THE BODY GOD DESIGNED

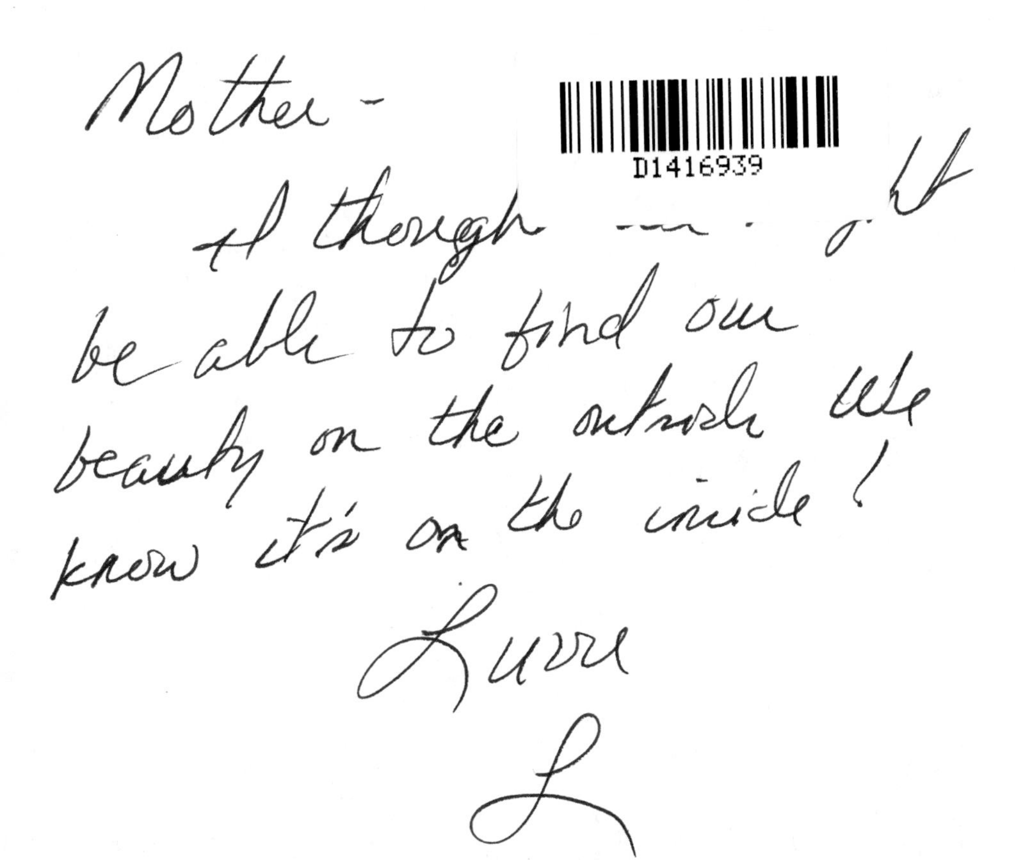

THE BODY GOD DESIGNED

GREGORY L. JANTZ, PhD

WITH ANN MCMURRAY

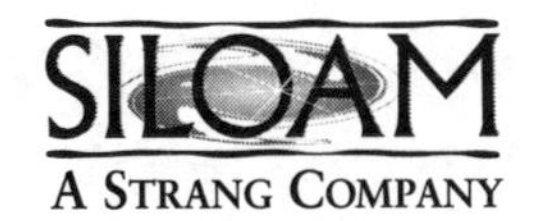

Most Strang Communications/Charisma House/Siloam/FrontLine/Excel Books/Realms products are available at special quantity discounts for bulk purchase for sales promotions, premiums, fund-raising, and educational needs. For details, write Strang Communications/Charisma House/Siloam/FrontLine/Excel Books/Realms, 600 Rinehart Road, Lake Mary, Florida 32746, or telephone (407) 333-0600.

The Body God Designed by Gregory L. Jantz, PhD, with Ann McMurray
Published by Siloam
A Strang Company
600 Rinehart Road
Lake Mary, Florida 32746
www.siloam.com

Cover Designer: Gearbox, studiogearbox.com
Executive Design Director: Bill Johnson

Library of Congress Cataloging-in-Publication Data:

Jantz, Gregory L.
The body God designed / Gregory L. Jantz ; with Ann McMurray.
p. cm.
Includes bibliographical references.
ISBN 978-1-59979-206-4
1. Weight loss--Religious aspects--Christianity. 2. Health--Religious aspects--Christianity. 3. Nutrition--Religious aspects--Christianity. I. McMurray, Ann. II. Title.

RM222.2.J367 2007
613.2'5--dc22

2007032424

08 09 10 11 12 — 9 8 7 6 5 4 3 2 1
Printed in the United States of America

Acknowledgments

I owe a very special debt of gratitude to my long-time collaborator, Ann McMurray, whose creativity, intelligence, and passion for the vision of The Center for Counseling and Health Resources (www.aplaceofhope.com) have been a constant source of inspiration for many.

Several colleagues read and made suggestions for this book, including the Center's clinic physician, Rhian Young, ND, whose solid whole-person approach provides great insights to those with stubborn weight struggles.

Our motto at the Center is, "Helping people change their lives for good." We acknowledge those lives in these pages, trusting that, with God, transformed lives are possible!

Contents

INTRODUCTION

God, When You Knit Me Together, You Dropped a Stitch

For you created my inmost being; you knit me together in my mother's womb. I praise you because I am fearfully and wonderfully made; your works are wonderful, I know that full well.

—Psalm 139:13–14

Many people look in the mirror and are dissatisfied with their bodies. Seat too big; chest too small. An enormous nose and beady eyes. Thunder thighs and bird legs. Ears that stick out and hair that sticks up. Psalm 139 says it's God's fault! Or is it? We get the "fearfully made" part; it's the "wonderfully made" we're not so sure about.

As we get started on this journey, where you're going to learn a bit about me and a lot more about yourself, allow me to confess a guilty pleasure. While waiting in the checkout line at the grocery store, I read magazine covers. And not just the "mainstream" ones like *People* or *Us*. I also read the tabloids. Yes, I know I shouldn't; I know they're not true, but, still, there's nothing else to do while waiting there, so I read them. How else would I know that Elvis has come back as an alien or somewhere in the world a woman has delivered a thirty-pound baby who looks like Winston Churchill?

The other day, I noticed a tabloid cover that spoke about exactly what we're going to discuss here. It was a story about how even movie stars have cellulite, complete with pictures of dimpled thighs and rears in tiny bathing suits. And just so you could *really* see that unsightly fat, there was a blown-up picture set in the larger one that showed only the offending back of a thigh. Glancing over at this cover, I had a kind of good-news/bad-news moment. On one hand, I felt perverse pleasure that even the tanned, muscled bodies of movie stars contend with cellulite. On the other hand, I was slightly depressed that even the tanned, muscled bodies of movie stars contend with cellulite. If their bodies aren't perfect, with all they do to maintain them, well, mine doesn't stand a chance. So, with a heavy heart, I paid for my Cinnabons and went home.

I don't figure we're too different, you and I. We care about our physical appearance. We want to look "good." Most of us are convinced we look "bad." Even if we're pleased with our overall appearance, there's always *something* we wish was different. Our desire to be perceived as attractive—inside and out—is fortified in so many ways: societal pressures, cultural standards, personal vanity, and personal insecurities. Somewhere along the line, we've developed a mental picture of not only what the perfect body should be but also what our own bodies would look like if they were perfect. Every time we look in the mirror, we experience a type of double vision. We see how we look at that moment, but we also perceive that ghost image of what we're *supposed* to look like, what we *would* look like if a variety of unfortunate features weren't there.

Add a Christian perspective to this dissatisfaction, and how we think about ourselves becomes complicated. After all, as Christians, we believe in Scripture. For example, in Matthew 5:48 Jesus says, "Be perfect, therefore, as your heavenly Father is perfect." We translate that perfection into not only spiritual characteristics but also physical ones. As Christians, providing a testimony to the rest of the world of the benefits of living a kingdom life, we truly believe we should be exemplary—exemplary in our relationships, exemplary in our personal habits, exemplary in our spiritual discipline, and exemplary in our physical appearance. Frankly, it's a lot of pressure. While we tend to effectively camouflage deficiencies in the other areas, it's pretty hard to hide our physical imperfections. Oh, not that we don't try.

In this age of medical marvels and surgical interventions, we've found another avenue to reach this elusive state of physical perfection, one where our inner image of our perfect self falls more in line with how we actually look. Seat too big? Have a butt tuck. Chest too small? Think breast augmentation. Prominent proboscis? A button nose is just a procedure and a couple weeks of recovery away. Poochy tummy? Liposuction. Wrinkles? Botox. Bird legs? Calf implants. Gray hair? Grecian Formula or L'Oreal. Receding hair? Plugs. Technology and advertising have an answer for everything, but is this really the way to achieve that perfect body?

What *is* a perfect body? Who determines what perfection looks like? Until now, we've allowed the superficial sciences (media in all forms) to specify who looks good and why. Not only does this practically perfect image become harder and harder to achieve (think Marilyn Monroe in the 1950s versus Kate Moss in the 1990s), but also it lasts only for a short window of time in your life. Older people in our society don't merely look good; they look good *at* forty or fifty or sixty. It's just our culture's way of saying, "Wow, you look pretty good...for an old person!" We're given a rigid standard of beauty that can only be achieved within an incredibly compressed timeline. This tyranny has to stop! People, Christians included, spend far too many hours agonizing over their bodies. It's time to stop longing for a perfect body and start recognizing and recovering, with God's help, the body God designed.

Rededicating the Temple

I love holidays, especially the New Year. It's a time to rededicate, to start anew. For many Christians, it's a time to commit to reading the Bible through during the year. Knowing and understanding Scripture is an excellent thing to do. Of course, reading the Bible through means actually reading the parts we tend to skim over at times. You know what parts I'm talking about—the genealogies (talk about mysteries—where do they come up with some of those names?), the instructions for the tabernacle in Exodus (carrying poles, basins, bases, rings, goat hair, fasteners, ephods, *whew!*), and all the rules and regulations in Leviticus (some of the most graphic and, frankly, weirdest parts of Scripture). Woe to those who attempt to honor their Bible-reading commitment at the end of a long day, sitting in anything resembling a comfortable chair!

As I write this, we're just into a new year, and I'm reading, in Exodus, God's directions for setting up the tabernacle. A couple of things popped into my mind. One, of course, is that I should always read in the morning. The other is the care and attention to detail God outlined for the tabernacle. This was essentially a big tent in the desert, a big movable tent. It struck me that God, the Creator of the universe, would take the time to detail with such specificity how He wanted the tabernacle to be built, even down to what colors to use for the stitching and embroidery work. God envisioned and planned for the tabernacle, His temple, to be built in a very specific way, one that would be functional as well as beautiful.

"Why are we talking about temples?" you may ask. "I just want to lose fifty pounds." Well, do you know your body is a temple? First Corinthians 6:19 says, "Do you not know that your body is a temple of the Holy Spirit, who is in you, whom you have received from God? You are not your own." Why are we talking about this? There's your answer: your body is a temple. God cared about the beauty and functionality of the Exodus tabernacle. He left very detailed instructions on how it should be built, moved, and maintained. He wanted it to become a focal point in the lives of His chosen people, Israel. By placing His presence inside the tabernacle, God granted a formerly enslaved, nomadic people the incredible honor and privilege of carrying around His presence and carrying out His will in the world.

So, what about your temple, your tabernacle? Do you think God is any less interested in your body? After all, your body is also a receptacle for His Spirit. By placing His presence in your body through the Holy Spirit, God is granting you, with all your faults and imperfections, the incredible honor and privilege of carrying around His presence and carrying out His will in the world. Instead of having one really big tabernacle to house His presence, God has allowed each one of us to act as a beautiful, functional, movable temple for His Spirit.

Please Pass the Guilt; I'd Like a Second Helping

Now, how's that for a load of guilt?

Before you beat yourself up any further for that Cinnabon desecrating God's temple, let's stop for a moment and gather some perspective. Yes, Psalm 139 says God created your body, that He knit it together. Scripture also says God knows even the number of hairs on your head (Matthew 10:30). So, God is responsible. He's responsible for the building blocks used to put your body together. You have a unique body given to you by God, ordained by Him even before the moment of conception. So, your small breasts and big hips are really God's fault. You have no control over your DNA. He's ultimately to blame for your thin legs and thinning hair. If you're unhappy with the way this body He's given you has turned out, God should accept responsibility and fix it, right?

It doesn't exactly work that way. Yet, some of us become quite angry with God if the latest diet doesn't work. We're genuinely miffed every time we look in the mirror and see those irritating imperfections. We think, "Why doesn't God help me change?" Or better yet, "Why doesn't God just change me?" The answer could be that God sees nothing wrong with the way He created you. The shape of your face or the size of your breasts may not be the current rage in this world, but that doesn't mean there's anything wrong with you. If you try to blame God for the foolish standard of worldly beauty and perfection, you're barking up the wrong tree.

What needs to change is not your body but your *perception* of your body. Perception is not reality. Your perception may say that your eyes are too narrow and your eyebrows too bushy. The reality is both your eyes and your eyebrows are functioning perfectly well, just as they're constructed to do. The "too" part comes from societal standards and has nothing to do with function and performance. Instead of praising God for the way in which He created your eyes and your eyebrows, you grumble and complain about "too" this and "too" that. Your perception leads to dissatisfaction. In that, you're joining a long line of grumblers and complainers, also known as the people of God whom Moses led out of captivity. Mad at God? Get in line.

I'm sure there were Israelites who really didn't like the way the tabernacle was constructed. Maybe they thought the carrying poles should be made of cedar and not acacia wood. Or maybe they thought silver rings were the way to go instead of gold or bronze. Or maybe they thought blue, purple, and scarlet yarn was so *yesterday*, so *Egypt*. Can you imagine God's reaction if someone had argued with Him over His instructions? Lightning bolts from the sky and being burned to a crisp come to mind. The sons of Aaron, Nadab and Abihu, come to mind. (Remember them? They were killed by God for offering a different kind of fire at the altar than He had prescribed. Simply put, they didn't follow instructions.)

Yet, don't we do the very same thing with God when it comes to our bodies? We're upset about the spacing of our eyes, the angle of our teeth, the length of our noses, and the size of our chests, bellies, and behinds. If our hair is naturally curly, we pay to have it straightened. If it's straight, we pay to have it curled. If it's brown, we color it or highlight it blonde. Instead of fighting God's design, we need to learn to operate within it to find all the beauty and functionality He's placed there. Instead of fighting against our own perceptions, we need to learn to accept our unique reality.

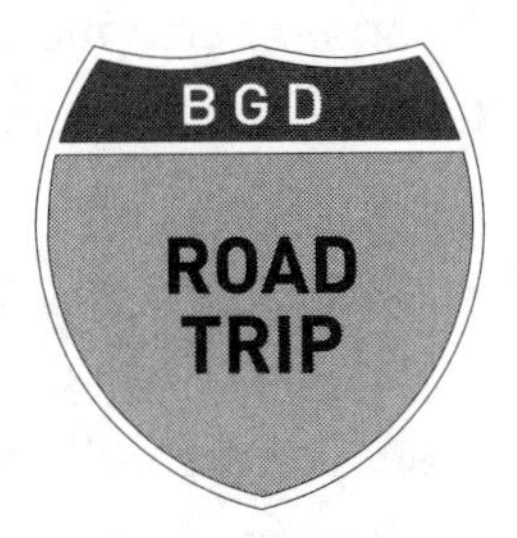

Every time you see this heading, know that I'm going to ask you to actually do something. It stands for "Body God Designed Road Trip," and each one will require you to get up, get active, and *do something*. This concept is very nicely outlined in

Proverbs 14:23, which says something to the effect that talk without action gets you nowhere. Just reading this book is not going to produce the body God designed for you by some sort of literary osmosis. This is not the equivalent of ruby slippers you can click together three times and say, "There's no place like home. There's no place like home. There's no place like home." To get to the "home" you seek, which is the body God designed for you, you're going to have to get up, move around, and take full advantage of the BGD Road Trips. Now, each BGD Road Trip may take you no farther than another part of your house or somewhere outside. (Remember, even in *The Wizard of Oz*, Dorothy learned her heart's desire was no farther than her own backyard because it was inside her all the time.)

Reading this book will help you understand a great deal about yourself and about God. But *understanding* is not enough; you also have to *act* upon that understanding. It's when you match your understanding to your action on a regular basis that you form a habit. Frankly, all of us have formed habitual ways of thinking about ourselves and our bodies based on all the wrong criteria and warped perceptions. BGD Road Trips are little actions you can take to help break up those habits so you can form new ones.

Enough reading for a bit. I'd like you to take a moment to think about your body. Recognizing that most of you still won't move from the spot where you are right now, nevertheless, I'm going to suggest that you get up off your rear and take this book into your bathroom or in front of a large mirror. Location-wise, you're probably not going very far. For some of you, however, just standing in front of a mirror and really looking at your body is like entering an entirely different dimension.

Oh, and make sure to pick up a pen and some paper on your way.

Are you in front of a mirror? OK, now, really look at yourself—from all angles. Look at every part of your body from the top of your head to the tips of your toes. What things just bug you about yourself? Write a list of all the aspects of your body (front, back, and sides) that distress you. If you could have any changes to your body right now, what would they be? You might say:

- "I wish I didn't have such a big mouth. When I smile, I look like the Cheshire cat from *Alice in Wonderland*."
- "I wish I had a full head of hair like when I was younger. Actually, better than when I was younger because even then it always looked weird."
- "I wish I could get rid of this baby fat. After all, this extra weight has been hanging around a long time—my babies are having babies."
- "I wish I could exchange the size of my waist for the size of my chest. Over the years, I've inverted."

If you frown, write it down! Whatever it is that causes you to frown when you look in the mirror, write it down, and then give your list this header:

Things I Really Don't Like About My Body

For some of you, I daresay this is the longest you've given yourself permission to look at your entire body in the mirror.

Usually, you try to whisk on past the mirror quickly, operating under the adage "Ignorance is bliss." However, for some of you, this kind of critical inspection is a normal part of your routine. Every time you're confronted with your image in any way, on any piece of glass, you use it as an opportunity to critically reflect on your reflection.

Were you able to come up with something to write down? Or did your hand cramp up after making all those tightly packed notations? However much you put down, it was pretty easy to find fault, wasn't it? You had no problem at all coming up with all the physical quirks that irritate you about your appearance. Being confronted by them every day makes them easy to remember.

Next, let's try something a little harder. Go back to that mirror, and write down all the things about your body or physical appearance you *do* like. What are your strong points? If you're having trouble coming up with any, I'll give you a hint: these will be things about your own body that you notice on the bodies of others. For example, if you see someone walking down the street and you say to yourself, "At least my ankles aren't as big as that woman's," or "I'm glad my gut isn't as out of shape as that guy's," these are the kinds of things to put on your list. They're the parts of your body or physical appearance you're least embarrassed about and might even, kind of begrudgingly, like. Head up this list with the words:

Things About My Body I'm Not Totally Disappointed With

(You'll notice that this list will be shorter than your first list. After all, why waste paper? I know at this stage it's easier to be critical than content. But take heart; that's what this book is about—helping you become less critical and more content with the body God created for you. So, be prepared for those lists to shift as we keep going.)

If you're really brave, you could do either of the following:

- Look at yourself without any clothing on. To really see your body, the one God created for you, the best way is "in the buff," not camouflaged by clothing. If this is difficult for you, ask for God to give you courage to look at yourself this way. God knows what you look like naked. He does not equate our nakedness with shame; that was our reaction, brought about by sin. Have courage and look at yourself as you truly are in the privacy of your own home and in the protection of God's acceptance and love.

- In order for you to do this next one, you'll need another person and probably some sort of legal waiver that you won't hold anything said against you by the other person for the next twenty years. But if you're brave and the other person is brave (and legally indemnified), have that brave someone you love write out all the things he or she finds wrong and finds right about your body, and then compare notes. You might find it interesting how your lists contrast and compare.

Now, look over the lists—"Things I Really Don't Like About My Body" and "Things About My Body I'm Not Totally Disappointed

With"—and on each list write down what is original equipment (OE) and what has been modified by the end user (EU—that would be you). Original equipment is how God made you. If you think your nose is too big or your eyes are too close together, that's original equipment. If you really dislike the shape of your hands or the cowlick on your head, that's original equipment. However, if you're irritated by the size of your tush or the way your thighs constantly rub together when you walk, that's an EU modification. God is not to blame that you're walking around in clothing three sizes too big that's still too tight.

"But wait," you say. "Aren't 'they' finding out there's a fat gene?" Nice try, but while some people do have different tendencies where weight gain and weight distribution are concerned, no one is doomed to obesity. We'll talk more about that later. For now, I want you to learn to accept those things about yourself that are a given and be alerted to those aspects about yourself that are subject to change. Think of this as your own Body Serenity Prayer:

> *God, grant me the serenity to accept the things about my body I cannot change, the courage to change the things I can for the better, and the wisdom to know the difference and get on with my life. Amen.*

That's basically what you're going to be doing with this book. You're going to really get to know your body and accept how God created each one of us in a different way. You're going to take a look again at the owner's manual (Scripture) for this original equipment that is your body and allow God to show you how to best care for and maintain it, even if it means making some personal changes. (You knew this part was going to be in here somewhere.) In the process, you're going to exchange a big helping of humble pie for a large dose of God's wisdom and perspective.

It's time to reorganize and rewrite your lists. I want you to take them both and categorize each item as either "Original Equipment" or "End-User Modification."

Keep these lists with this book. From this point on, you are going to use these lists for your personal prayer time and meditation on the journey to the body God designed for you. Next to "Original Equipment," I want you to write, "Blessings From God." As you write the words, the items you listed under "Original Equipment" will become more tangible as your personal blessings from God. "What?" you say. "How can I possibly consider my big nose a blessing?" It's a blessing because it's original equipment, the way God made you. Besides, who says it's big? Compared to what? Compared to whom? Somewhere, someone has told you your nose is big, and you've decided your nose is a negative. The negative here is *not* your nose; it's the snarky comment by that other person! Reject the comment, and learn to love your nose. It's unique, just like you. You don't have to be like everyone else to be beautiful. That's society talking, and it's time to tell it to be quiet! Say to yourself, "I love my nose, thank you! It's a gift from my Father."

Next to "End-User Modifications," I want you to write, "I'm committing these to God." Your "End-User Modifications" list is what you are going to commit to changing with God's help. For most of you, many of the items on this list are going to have a common denominator—excess weight. Welcome to our twenty-first-century culture. The wonderful thing is that by committing to work toward achieving and maintaining a healthy weight for yourself, you'll be working on multiple end-user modifications at once.

Give both of these lists to God. Thank Him for His original equipment and ask for His help on the end-user modifications. This endless battle of beauty and perfection is using up too many of the emotional, personal, and financial resources of God's people. It's time to accept God's direction for the building, maintenance, and movement of your body. After all, you need to get to the point in your life when you're able to redirect this inward focus and get on with the business of being God's presence in the world. No more navel gazing! There's a great big world out there with a lot of wonderful things to see, do, and be a part of. I don't know about you, but I'm ready to get started!

Father, I am fearfully and wonderfully made. Help my heart to know it and accept it in all the fullness You desire. Help me to be the very best I can be for You! Amen.

Chapter 1

I've Been Framed!

> My frame was not hidden from you when I was made in the secret place. When I was woven together in the depths of the earth, your eyes saw my unformed body.
>
> —Psalm 139:15–16

We look at supermodels and athletes in media and adopt their body shapes as our epitome of perfection. Surely this is what Adam and Eve looked like in the garden—tanned, muscled, voluptuous, virile. And just as happened to them, we've been cursed, all right, but with a body that will never boast a chiseled chest or a flat stomach. But what if God, in His wisdom, didn't set up one particular style of body as the model for us all? What if a model isn't supposed to be the model?

The Wisdom of the Ages

Let's stop and think for a moment about what beauty has meant over time and culture. Frankly, societal standards haven't been noted for tolerance and inclusion. Surely you remember seeing *National Geographic* pictures of tribal cultures in which beauty was defined as dinner-plate-sized lips (growing children have larger and larger plates inserted into their lips until it becomes virtually impossible to eat anything but liquids) or in which the signature attractive feature is an unnaturally elongated neck (rings encircling the necks of young children are added to each year until the bones of the neck are so long and fragile that if the rings are removed, it's life threatening). How about the physical beauty enhancement of body scarring (where the rough places that contrast so strikingly with the smooth skin actually started out as red, raw, intentional wounds to the body)? Or what about the ancient cultural practice of binding girls' feet to the point that they were effectively imprisoned in their own homes after they grew up, hardly able to hobble? Oh, yes, there's nothing like culture to come up with the concept of beauty, is there?

Now, you may argue that these examples are from barbaric or backward times and that we, as Americans awash in the dawn of the twenty-first century, are so much more culturally aware. Our societal standards of beauty make sense, unlike others. After all, our culture would never force such drastic definitions of beauty on anyone! *Hmmm*, is that really true though? What about young women—and more increasingly, young men—who purposely starve themselves of both food and fluids in order to achieve an ever-lowering target of ideal weight? How about a culture in which a portion of those chosen as representatives of physical beauty qualify as anorexic under diagnostic and medical criteria? Consider a culture so bulging with excess that people gorge themselves until bursting with food and then induce vomiting for fear of becoming fat. What about a society that places extreme value on the most fleeting characteristic of all, youth, and that defines worth, value, and beauty in such narrow terms that it consigns most of its people to a twilight, faded, left-behind status?

If I were writing this in an e-mail message, I'd start using CAPITAL LETTERS at this point. Doesn't what you've just read make you mad?

Aren't you angry at how you've been demoralized and devalued by societal standards? Don't you want to yell and scream in rage at this artificial standard that passes you by so quickly you spend your youth reaching for it, only to find it rushes by, out of your grasp, as you age? Are you angry enough to let it go? In order for you to appreciate a body of God's design, you must jettison the chains of worldly perceptions so you'll be free to accept God's truth about who you are and how valuable you are.

God is not bound to the latest iterations of physical perfection, nor does He consider His only recent successes to be Angelina Jolie or Brad Pitt. (I use those names with hesitation, realizing that even mentioning them will "date" this book. The dubious honor of being one of the current "beautiful people" has the shelf life of an in-use cell phone.) Cultural standards have handed us a gift akin to the unwelcome Christmas present you receive each year from your Aunt Minnie in Duluth. It's a "one-size-fits-all" standard of beauty. I don't know about you, but when I put this "gift" on, it doesn't fit, no matter what the label says. There are parts of me that stick out and stretch and other parts that look shrunken and baggy. Thanks, but no thanks. I'm tired of listening to what the world has to say about my body. I'm ready to start listening to God.

Have you noticed that God seems to enjoy diversity? Look at flowers: they come in virtually any size, shape, and color. From tiny alpine meadow blossoms to enormous, spiky dahlias, from the simplicity of a daisy to the extravagance of an orchid, from the palest of yellows to almost black reds, flowers certainly speak to God's creative genius and preference for variety. Why, then, do we accept God's design for flowers but not His design for people? It's as if we look out over a vast array of thousands of blooms and decide we'll only be happy if given just one—that one way over there in the left-hand corner that you can barely see and can't get to easily; and it doesn't matter if there's one two feet away that's very much like it. It has to be *that* one way over there or nothing!

We've just had a Toys "R" Us toddler moment. If any of you have taken a toddler to Toys "R" Us, you know exactly what I mean! We are pitching a societal temper tantrum against God because of our unhappiness about our bodies! I think it's time we grew up and moved on. After all, as much as God loves His flowers, He loves us more: "Consider how the lilies grow. They do not labor or spin. Yet I tell you, not even Solomon in all his splendor was dressed like one of these. If that is how God clothes the grass of the field, which is here today, and tomorrow is thrown into the fire, how much more will he clothe you, O you of little faith!" (Luke 12:27–28). God has clothed us in the body He's provided, which, like field grass, isn't slated to last long. Just as God enjoys and has a purpose for each flower He creates, no matter how long it lives, God enjoys and has a purpose for each *person* He creates, no matter how long he or she is on the earth. He clothes that flower or that person in an earthly body. For God, there is no one-flower-type-fits-all. In the same way, for Him there is no one-body-type-fits-all. Let's take a look at the diversity of these earthly bodies and learn to appreciate the beauty in each.

Across the Fruited Plain

Body shapes are fascinating. Have you ever taken a break at a busy shopping mall or amusement park, or street corner for that matter, and just watched people? Every body is different, but there are similarities. Popular wisdom has defined these similarities in the form of fruit—most of us have apple, pear, or banana bodies. And, naturally for popular wisdom, these fruit shapes are categorized by how each shape carries fat. In today's culture, there's just no getting around this obsession with fat (we'll get into it more in chapter 5), but these categories do have some value, so let's take a look at them.

Banana people (also known as sticks or runner beans, go figure) don't have any excess fat. In fact, it's hard for this body type to gain either weight or muscle. They are just lean people who seem to be able to eat what they want, when they want. Bananas don't have much curve to them at all; they tend to have little difference between chest, waist, and hip (prior to plastic surgery, at least). Many people envy bananas because they seem to have won the genetic lottery where potlucks are concerned.

Apple people are those who carry most of their weight around their middles. They've got normal-sized arms and legs but tend to be excessively round around their chests and stomachs. Apples are the inner-tube people, with their fat around their middles.

Pear people are those who carry their weight below their waist in their hips and thighs. It's as if an apple person took that inner-tube of fat and shoved it down around his hips and bottom. Pears have normal-sized chests and waists, but their hips are wider than their shoulders.

I think women must have come up with these fruit analogies. Men tend to classify body shapes not around fat but around muscularity. For men, fruit is out; morphs are in.

Ectomorphs are thin guys who can't seem to bulk up, even when they work out. *Endomorphs* are guys who don't or won't work out, basically couch potatoes or, better yet, couch apples or couch pears. In the male lottery of life, the *mesomorphs* are the ones who hit the jackpot with athletic, hard bodies.

For women, thin is in; for men, bulk is best. Or is it? Even within these different body shapes, there are pluses and minuses. So, don't gloat or despair! Understand your body type and what to watch out for.

Banana health

Let's look at bananas first. These can translate into ectomorphs, for the sake of grouping. While it is true that these individuals are thin, they are also not naturally powerful. They can, however, exchange power for stamina with the right training. A healthy banana or ectomorph is able to stick with a task over the long term. Slow and steady wins the race for these fairly rare people. If you are a banana, you should watch for:

- Using your natural thinness as an excuse to eat whatever you want. It's still important to eat a healthy choice of food, especially protein to maximize lean muscle production.
- Adopting a sedentary lifestyle and risking osteoporosis in later years. Thin and wispy as a young adult can translate into frail and weak in old age.
- Not interpreting outer thinness for inner health. No matter what your body shape, it is important to know your inner health factors, such as overall cholesterol, HDL and LDL cholesterol, triglyceride levels, blood pressure, and heart rate.

Apple health

Apples, and those endomorphs with an apple shape, have big bellies, true, but they still have thin arms and legs. They put on weight more quickly but also can drop weight more quickly than pears. With a drop in weight, apples lose fat around their middles and can alter how they look and their health profile. If you are an apple, you should watch for:

- Excessive weight around your middle. This outer fat can point to inner fat known as intra-abdominal fat, which wraps itself around internal organs, such as the heart.

- Developing high-risk conditions, such as heart disease, stroke, diabetes, gallbladder problems, and hypertension because of the presence of this intra-abdominal fat.

Pear health

Pears, and those endomorphs who adopt a pear shape, appear to be less at risk for the conditions listed above. Their fat is much lower in their bodies at the hips and thighs and farther away from vital organs. When pears lose weight, however, they tend to lose more in the upper body than the lower body, maintaining their pear shape. They merely become smaller pears. If you are a pear, you should watch for:

- Excessive dieting to try and change your basic shape. Your main fat-storage areas are in the hips and thighs, and that will not change.
- Becoming discouraged and giving up on healthy eating, figuring that if you're still going to have thunder thighs, you might as well go ahead and have that Snickers bar.

Now, mesomorphs—or the highly muscled people—also have a caution. Young mesomorphs tend to become old endomorphs unless they keep up with a fitness program. Think of your thirty-year high school reunion. Some of those star athletes will have magically transformed into plump middle-agers. While your body may have a genetic predisposition to lean muscle, it won't just appear or remain without diligence, healthy eating, and an active lifestyle. What was a given in high school can slowly be taken away by middle age.

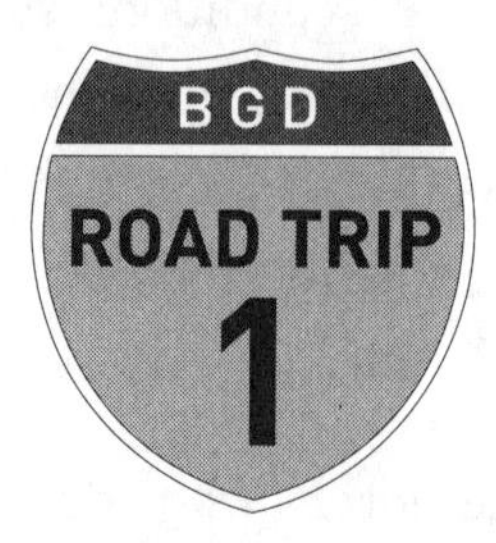

It's time to take stock of your body shape. So it's time for a road trip. This time, you'll need to travel wherever there's a mirror, and make sure to pick up a measuring tape on your way. Oh, and if it's been awhile since you did any math, grab a calculator, too.

There are some pretty good health reasons to determine what your shape is, especially when it comes to being either an apple or a pear. Apples have heightened health risks, so you want to know where you fall. (It would be the apple that leads to the fall.) One of the quickest ways to tell if you're an apple or a pear is to look in the mirror. Stand relaxed in front of the mirror with your arms at your side. If your arms and legs are relatively normal but the bulk of your excess weight is riding around your middle, you're an apple. If your bulk is centered south of the border, you're a pear. Here's another way to tell: check your waist-to-hip ratio (this is where the calculator comes in).

If you're a man:

- Measure your waist at your navel.
- Measure your hips at the tip of the hip bone.

If you're a woman:

- Measure your waist right at the base of your ribs.

- Measure your hips at the widest part of your hips and buttocks.

To find your waist-to-hip ratio (WHR):

- Divide your waist size by your hip size.
- Ideally, your WHR should be 0.80 or less if you're a woman.
- Ideally, your WHR should be 0.95 or less if you're a man.
- If your WHR is more than these, you are, or are becoming, an apple.

Fruit of the Spirit

Now before you pears and bananas figure you're off the hook, please remember the name of this book—*The Body God Designed*. Remember, we're talking about the body that God gave you when you were formed. These earthly definitions are of some value, but they must not overshadow God. If your body tends toward being an apple, there's nothing wrong with you! And if you have a banana body, you're not inherently righteous! These are things to keep track of and factor in, but they do not define your value to God. He gave you your body, and He wasn't having a bad day at the moment of your conception.

For some of us, we have no idea what the body God gave us should look like. Sometimes our bodies are altered through the circumstances of life. Accidents happen. Illness occurs. We exist in a fallen world, and that's just part of the landscape we live in. More than we care to admit, we may have altered our bodies with our lifestyle choices to the point that they resemble more an expression of our will than God's. We decide to smoke, to drink too much, to eat too much, to worry too much, to work too much, to eat too little, to relax too little, to move too little. With these choices, we compromise the health God has given us, and we alter the body He designed.

One of the greatest dangers to the body God designed for you is excess weight. This burden of pounds wears out your joints. It strains your heart. It jumbles your hormonal system. It suffocates your breathing. It diverts your thoughts. Excess weight and obesity are like insistent squatters who never go home, always demanding your time, attention, and energy. If your body is a temple, obesity and excess weight are like money changers, taking up residence for their own reasons apart from God (John 2:13–16). Jesus chased those money changers out with a whip (Matthew 21:12); you need to do the same with yours. Obesity and excess weight must be evicted from your temple to reclaim God's promise of health.

One great thing about God is it's never too late to start again. If you've altered your body to the point you don't know where your alterations end and God's design begins, you can commit right now to making positive changes to recapture His unique gift. (Remember, it's *your* body I'm talking about, not someone else's. You cannot demand that God give you Angelina Jolie's or Brad Pitt's body. Don't be like the Toys "R" Us toddler who throws down his own present and tries to snatch away the gift of another. When you do that, you tell God you don't appreciate the body He's given especially to you.)

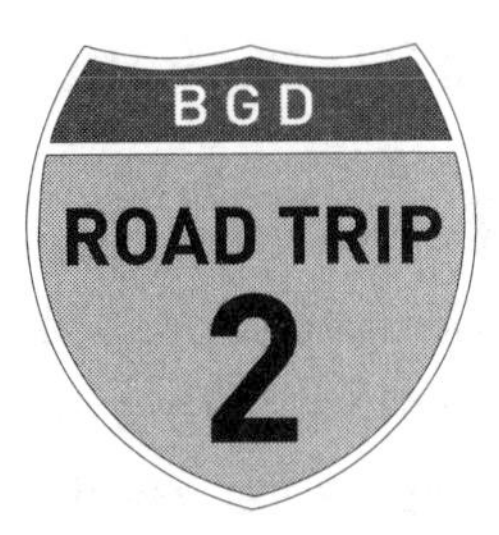

This road trip is going to take you to the far-off regions of your bedroom closet. Whatever your shape is now, you need to accept it. Pretending you're a size eight when you're really a size fourteen, or a size thirty-two when you're really a forty-two, isn't going to help. Thinking you can change overnight from a size fourteen to a size eight, or from a size forty-two to a size thirty-two, won't help either. It's time to clean house! Clear out those thoughts, and clear out those clothes! Now, you know what clothes I mean—those surely-I'll-be-able-to-wear-this-someday clothes.

It's kind of interesting how those surely-I'll-be-able-to-wear-this-someday clothes got to be in your closet. For guys, often these are the clothes you wore when you were younger—and smaller. You keep them around, just on the off-chance that lightning should strike and you wake up one day twenty pounds lighter. They're old and worn, but you have high hopes one day you'll be able to fit into them again and recapture just a little bit of your younger, thinner days. Now, women seem to have some of these surely-I'll-be-able-to-wear-this-someday clothes that are old, but more often they have clothes that are new. This represents their forward-thinking delusion that says, "If I just have this size in my closet, I'm destined to become it someday. In fact, the more I have of a certain size, the greater the critical mass generated to produce a resulting drop in weight." (I'm sure there's a mathematical formula involved here, although I have no idea what it is.)

Enough of this! I want you to go up to your room and clear out all those clothes. Go up to your closet and your drawers and clean house! Keep only those clothes that *actually* fit you. If you have something of sentimental value, go ahead and keep it, but wrap it in plastic and put it in a box under a bed in some other room. Be honest. Go through every piece of clothing you own, *including underwear*. If it doesn't fit, don't wear it. If you don't have enough clothes left that actually fit, go shopping. If money is tight, go to a consignment or thrift store. (Be aware, however, you'll have to fight off the high school and college kids who tend to frequent these stores looking for bargains. Don't think of going to a thrift store as a financial necessity; consider it *trendy*.)

If you need more underwear, start there. Underwear is the article of clothing worn closest to your body. The tighter they are, the more folds and indentations they make; the more they pinch in, the more other things pooch out. When these items fit correctly, they help the rest of your clothes hang correctly. Buying the correct size underwear is a huge step in the right direction of accepting your body the way it is right now. Accepting your body right now helps you to feel good about yourself.

It's difficult to make positive changes if you don't feel good about yourself. It's hard to feel good about yourself if your clothes don't fit. Stop jamming yourself into too-tight jeans. Remove any shirts that must stretch to triple their size when you wear them. If zippers snag and buttons pop, if pants ride up and jackets don't meet, bid them a fond farewell. You're about to enter the realm of reality. This is who—and how big—you are now.

Putting Things Into Proportion

Are you feeling lousy because this field trip to your own room has reminded you of how much weight you've gained? Did you become so focused on your outward appearance that you forgot that God cares about your inner qualities? In all that activity, did you forget God loves you? He also loves courage and truth. It takes courage to accept the truth of how things are right now. You've gotten out of "shape"; that's true. You know what's also true? God can help you recover your true shape again. He can help you become healthier than you've ever been, no matter your age.

Today, be happy with who you are. Are you perfect? No? Well, who is? Remember, even those muscled, tanned movie stars have cellulite. Why? Because even muscled, tanned movie stars did something wrong? No. Because cellulite is a natural condition of the human body. It's not evil or ugly; it's normal. Our healthy bodies are made by God to contain a certain amount of stored fat. Everyone's body will place those stores in genetically designed places. When God considers the worth of a person, believe me, He doesn't make value judgments based upon deposits of subcutaneous fat. It's the world's job to make shallow and superficial judgments like that.

Instead of concentrating your efforts on what you see as wrong with you, focus your energies on what you can do to make things right today and tomorrow. Your body is an amazing piece of work. (Now, don't go saying to yourself, "I know. That's why I'm reading this book—because I'm such a piece of work!") Whatever your shape, your body is designed with an amazing ability to heal, to correct, to generate health. Working with your body and its God-designed systems, you can get back into shape, and I don't mean some idealized, impossible shape, but the very shape God intended when He created you.

I think it's easier to remember things if you can put them into recognizable, memorable phrases. A common thread in this chapter has been accepting who God made you to be and where you are right now. To me, that's the foundation of rediscovering your body the way God designed it. You must first **(A)—Accept yourself**. If you don't accept who you are right now, if you resent or hate yourself, it's going to be very difficult to find the positive motivation you need to move forward. From now on, you must daily remind yourself to *accept yourself*. You are not allowed to beat yourself up anymore! Can you learn lessons and gain wisdom from your past? Absolutely! But you must look at yourself, as God does, with new compassion every single day, just as Lamentations 3:22–23 says. God, even knowing all He does about your past, your present, and your future, daily has compassion for you. If He can do that, you can at least accept yourself each day. This positive acceptance can power your motivation to change. It's kind of a paradox, really, which seems to be God's stock-in-trade, but by accepting yourself today, you find the strength to change yourself for tomorrow.

Father, help me to live in the reality of this moment and accept the truth about myself. Guard me from self-hatred, and teach me to love myself as You love me. Allow this love for who You are, who I am, and who You created me to be, to motivate me today to love myself more. Today I need the reality of Your love to replace the perceptions of this world. Amen.

CHAPTER 2

HINT: THE GARDEN WAS OUTDOORS

> Now the Lord God had planted a garden in the east, in Eden; and there he put the man he had formed.
>
> —GENESIS 2:8

God didn't create Adam and Eve to live in a condo in the midst of a bustling urban metropolis. Rather, He placed them in a garden—outdoors. He gave them the physically challenging work of tending the garden. In other words, God made us to be physically active. We were made for handling a hoe, not a remote. Could that be why our bodies respond positively to rigorous physical activity?

From Tilling Potatoes to Being One

OK, let's think about a typical day for many average Americans. We get out of bed in the morning, move around a little to get ready, grab some breakfast and the paper, and sit down to eat and read. Then we move around a little bit more, at least enough to get out the door and into our cars, so we can sit in our cars to get to work. Then we move a little to get to work so we can sit a long time at our desks. We may move around a little while there, but mostly we're sitting until we move around a little so we can leave—to get into our cars and sit on the way home. Once home, we sit down to have dinner and sit down to watch *American Idol.* We move around a little to get ourselves to bed, where we sleep until we get up and do it all again the next day. Each day, we move around a little and sit a whole lot more. And, somehow, in the midst of all of this, we think we're going to lose weight. This is not defined as logic but as wishful thinking.

Our brave new world is a long way from Eden. We've gone from tilling potatoes to being one—of the variety *couchum sedentarii.*

The Parking Lot Syndrome

OK, here's another example. We're in our cars (again) and driving to—well, you fill in the blank. Pulling into the parking lot, our senses are heightened as we circle like vultures for that one prime parking spot. In the grips of primal hunting behavior, we're looking for the one that's the absolute closest to the entrance. We spend ten minutes circling, hovering, positioning our car, in order to park thirty feet from the building instead of one hundred thirty feet. Of course, if we'd just parked in the first empty parking space we saw driving in, we could have walked that extra one hundred feet in a matter of seconds, but that's not really the point. Or is it?

Not Even Remotely Physical

OK, last example. Now you're in your recliner or on your couch watching television—at night after a large meal on a day when you haven't really moved much at all—and you realize you want to change the channel. The television is probably eight or ten feet away. What's the first thing you do? Get up and change the channel? No way! That's so 1950s! The first thing you do is look for the remote. If you're a woman, you may first have to pry it away from whatever male inhabits your house. If you're a man, you've probably got it within arm's reach, if you're not clutching it automatically.

You get the remote so you don't have to move to get up. (However, you will move to *find* the remote. But you won't move to change the channel—go figure.) We've arrived at this grand juncture in history where it is now an *imposition* to have to physically move yourself ten feet.

And it's not remotes for just the television anymore. There are remotes for a whole plethora of electronic devices—stereos, coffee-pots, DVD players. There are "clap on/clap off" devices so you don't even have to go to the effort of turning a knob or flipping a switch or pushing a button. This last modern marvel always reminds me of one of those old Hollywood movies set in cheesy desert Kasbah with a corpulent potentate who merely has to clap his hands to make his servants jump to accommodate his every wish. When did "clap on/clap off" become our idea of paradise?

The lesson of the remote? We're not even remotely physical anymore.

Sweatin' to the Oldies

So, when did we all come to this subconscious decision as a culture that physical movement was an imposition? When did we decide that getting up to change the channel or turn off a light was a monumental waste of time and effort? We may have done this to ourselves incrementally, under the category of unintended consequences. In searching for ways to make our lives more convenient, we've made them less physical. Why? Because physical work is hard; it involves sweat and effort and, in some cases, aches and pains. In some other cases, physical work, frankly, is dangerous. I think we started out trying to make our lives less physical in order to make them less dangerous. Then we morphed from avoiding physically dangerous work to avoiding physical work in general. Some of us are so far now from tending a garden that we can't even keep a houseplant alive.

Of course, part of this might be simple rebellion—rebellion to something that started long, long ago in a garden far, far away. Let's go back to that garden, to the third chapter of Genesis. This is the chapter where all hell breaks loose, literally. Eve is tempted by the forbidden fruit and buys the serpent's lie that God really doesn't mean what He says. Not wanting to take the blame alone, she gets Adam to join her in sin, and then they both do what we normally do when we mess up—they tried to hide it. God, of course, knows exactly where they are and what they've done, but He wants them to confess anyway. Which they do—kind of—at the end of chapter 3, and then God explains the consequences of their actions. One of these consequences involves the curse of physical labor. He even mentions the word *sweat*. It has a very negative connotation.

Most of us don't like sweat. It's sticky; it's smelly; it's unsightly. It means we've been working hard and exerting physical effort, which we also do our very best to avoid. We don't like it. Yet God says we're destined for it because of our sin. He says because of our sin we're going to have to toil by the sweat of our brow because work is now going to be a whole lot harder. The cushy garden job is no longer available, and every other job is a whole lot higher on the sweat-o-meter. We really don't like sweat now; it's part of our curse.

Do you know the word translated as "sweat" appears only twice in the whole Bible? It appears once in the Old Testament and once in the New Testament. In the Old Testament, God says sweat is our lot now because of sin. Can you guess who is mentioned in connection with sweat in the New Testament? You're right; the only other time sweat is mentioned is in regards to Jesus. Luke 22:44 says, "And being in anguish, he prayed more earnestly, and his sweat was like drops of blood falling to the ground." And where was Jesus when He was sweating? In another garden. Full circle.

Jesus wasn't afraid to sweat. He was willing to sweat for us. Sweat was a curse in one garden and an act of redemption in another. I think it's time to stop looking at sweat as a curse and try to claim its redemptive nature. It's time to stop thinking of sweat as something bad and begin to understand it as something good for the body God designed.

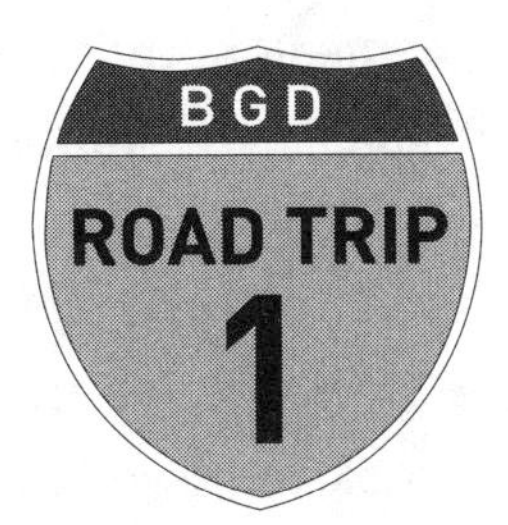

Before we go any further, however, it's time to get up and move around; it's time for your first BGD Road Trip of this chapter. You're going to go into several rooms in your house and list all of the ways you have minimized the need for physical movement during your day. Keep your eyes open, and think about how you use each room as you look at it. Following are some things to think about, but they are by no means meant to substitute for your list. I offer them just to get your mental juices flowing and to help you see where I'm going with this:

- Family room—This could be called a den or TV room. Do you have a remote for your television? Your stereo? What about the placement of the couch or chair? Have you positioned your furniture to make it more convenient to sit and watch television? What is the focal point of the room? Is this room where your computer is? How much time do you spend in this room? Have you substituted outdoor, physical activity time for time in front of the television or on the computer?

- Kitchen—Have you set up your kitchen to be one of convenience? What part of your refrigerator is used the most, the refrigerator or the freezer? Are your meals nutritious? Convenient? Are they meant to take the shortest amount of time to prepare even if they aren't the best for you? Which is used more: the stove and oven or the microwave? Do you move around the space to prepare and cook, or do you dash in and out as quickly as possible just to get food on the table? Do you eat meals while watching television? Do you eat in general while watching television?

- Bedroom—How much time do you spend here? Is this room used as a place to rejuvenate for the next day? Is there a television in your bedroom? Do you spend time lying in bed and watching TV? What about a computer? Do you take your laptop to bed with you? Do you have a device on your lights so you don't have to get up out of bed to turn them off? How close is your alarm clock to your bed? Do you have to get up out of bed in the morning to turn it off, or is it right next to you, where you can hit the snooze bar repeatedly just by flopping your arm?

- Spare bedroom—In my house this is also known as the junk room. If it's been awhile since you've been in this room, or if it's inconvenient for you to even occasionally pass through all the rooms in your house, that's probably a red flag. If you have been in this room lately, has it been to spend some time moving things around to organize and clean? Or was it just long enough to open the door and fling some unwanted-at-the-moment item onto the nearest surface?

- Garage—This is a big one. It's probably where you have your car (although it also could be parked outside because of all of the stuff in here). The car is one of the greatest ways we've reduced our need to move physically. Like many great inventions, it's both a blessing and a curse. How do you use your car? Will you drive five blocks to take your child to school instead of walking? Go back to the parking lot scenario. Do you tend to use your car to get the closest you can to your destination? Do you consider it a failure on your part to have to settle for an outlying parking spot? Let's go back to the garden. What about any garden tools? Is your grass the size of a postage stamp but you have a gas-powered mower anyway? Do you have powered edgers and clippers? Do you even have yard tools, or does someone else physically take care of your yard? Do you even have a yard?

- Stairs—Do you have stairs in your house? What about stairs to get into your house or condo or apartment? What about stairs in general? Do you try to avoid them at any cost? In stores, hotels, or airports, will you use an elevator or an escalator to avoid stairs? When you're at home, do you create a pile at the bottom of the stairs so you only have to make one trip up instead of multiple ones? Do you ask your spouse or your kids to get you something from upstairs (if you're downstairs) or downstairs (if you're upstairs) in order to avoid using the stairs yourself? When you chose where to live, did you partly do so because of the lack of stairs?

Most of us don't make a conscious decision to be sedentary. Rather, our sedentary lifestyles develop through the thousands of little decisions we make each day. Hopefully, this road trip will help you to see the impact of all of your little decisions on how physically active you are just where your home is concerned.

I didn't have you do all of that to make you depressed about what a couch potato you've become. (And please tell me you actually *did* get up out of your chair to do it. If you haven't yet, if you're still just sitting there reading, it's not too late. Get up and do it! Then come back. The book's not going anywhere.) I had you do that to empower you through knowledge. When you understand what you're doing, you're better prepared to do something different, because, frankly, if you're going to attain the body God designed for you, you're going to have to do something different. Different doesn't have to be bad or scary, though it will be sweaty, but that's OK.

A Stitch in Time Saves Nine

Before I get into all of the wonderful, glorious benefits of physical exercise, I have one more misnomer I want you to recognize so you can let go of it and jettison it from your thinking. This is an "out with the old, in with the new" kind of thing. I've talked about the unintended consequences of our thirst for convenience. I've talked about our rebellion against anything that requires a great deal of physical effort. Let's talk about our love affair with time.

In this culture, time is the new currency. Physical effort takes time. It takes time to walk instead of drive. It takes time to get up and turn on a light instead of clapping our hands. It takes time to exercise. Most people I know want to be more physically active; the problem they have is with time. They don't think they have the time to exercise. They haven't found the right time. There isn't enough time in the day, they tell me.

After all, we live in a time-compressed, do-it-now, too-much-to-do-in-too-little-time world. We're constantly looking for ways to get more time out of our days. That's why cell phones are so amazingly popular. I cannot imagine what I did before without the ability to use all of that commuting time as work time by using my cell phone. Sometimes, I feel guilty actually listening to music or having a quiet moment in the car when I could be on my cell phone taking care of one more urgent item.

I think if you asked a large cross section of Americans what they'd rather have more of—money or time—you may be surprised at how many say time. That's why I think time is the new currency. And we've decided that physical activity is not something we want to spend that money (time) on. We'd rather spend it on all the urgent, pressing matters in our days until we're so exhausted that we have no time left and nothing left to give physically.

This is where the good news comes in. Your body, as I said before, was created by God to operate as a physical being. You're not just made to operate physically; you're made to operate *better* physically. Physical exercise doesn't just spend your currency of time; it actually pays dividends.

Sweat Equity

If you google "benefits of physical exercise," you'll get over five *million* responses. The fact that physical exercise is good for the body is not a secret. Here are just a few of the known benefits, which increase almost on a daily basis as more research is done:

- Increased flexibility
- Stronger muscles
- Increased bone density
- Increased stamina and endurance
- Lower risk of coronary artery disease
- Lower blood pressure

- Higher levels of good cholesterol and lower levels of bad cholesterol
- Helps control blood lipid abnormalities (that's from the American Heart Association)
- Helps control diabetes
- Helps control obesity
- Better survival rates for those who have suffered a heart attack
- Improved mood; lessened depression
- Improved quality of life
- Stress relief
- Better sleep
- Increased metabolism
- Stronger immune system
- Positive benefits even with moderate changes in exercise level

If you could take a pill that would give you all those benefits, would you take it? Of course you would! If you weighed all these benefits against the time it takes to pop a pill, there's no comparison. But what if you weighed the benefits of physical activity against the time it takes to *be* physically active? Not quite as much of a slam dunk, is it? That's because you're still weighed down with your attitudes about convenience, time, and sweat. Exercise is inconvenient; it takes time, and you sweat when you do it. For many of us, that just tipped the scales back in the direction of *why bother*. But by tipping the scales in that direction, you've just sent your bathroom scales and your body designed by God in the wrong direction.

The Journey of One Thousand Miles

Do you know that adage that says something like, "The journey of one thousand miles starts with a single step"? The basic premise is you can go a long way over time if you do small things today. I put it a different way. There's a term I use that's very helpful to me personally and to those I counsel with. It's the term *baby steps*. (I think I came up with this term even before Bill Murray's character in *What About Bob?*) In therapy, baby steps are the small increments (steps) of simple, doable (baby) things that a person can do to get better. They are realistic and attainable. Not single steps *of* one thousand miles but single steps *toward* one thousand miles. Baby steps are the way you change your habits and your life slowly and steadily.

The world says you have to take thousand-mile leaps in order to be successful. God knows better. He knows we learn incrementally and that understanding is a journey. In Romans 12:2, Paul talks about this incremental change when he says, "And do not be conformed to this world, but be transformed by the renewing of your mind, so that you may prove what the will of God is, that which is good and acceptable and perfect" (NASU). He doesn't say your mind will be—*ZAP*—transformed in one fell swoop. He says transformation is a process and renewal is a life journey. After all, it was God who sent His people on a little journey for forty years in the wilderness, truly a thousand-mile journey made up of single steps. Was all that wandering a waste of time? No. During the journey the people of Israel learned about God, and they learned about themselves. Similarly, in order to achieve your thousand-mile destination, your body designed by God, you need to accept that you're on a journey. The journey itself is not a waste of time because along the way you're going to learn about God, and you're going to learn about yourself. Do not despise God because He's asking you to take baby steps toward your destination instead of miraculously transporting you there in one fell swoop.

Too often we focus on the destination and not the journey. "One thousand miles!" you say. "That's too much!" It's not as much as you think. I run an average of twenty miles per week. At the end of the year, that's just over one thousand miles. And how do I run those one thousand miles? One step at a time. It's not my "goal" to run one thousand miles a year. Rather, my goal is to get outside, enjoy the day, and get some physical exercise. The one thousand miles is a result of something I enjoy doing. Your own journey of one thousand miles can also be the result of something you enjoy doing.

Wait. I know what some of you are going to say: "But I *enjoy* sitting and watching television." True; so do I, but that's not the *only* thing I enjoy doing. The good news is you can take those baby steps along your journey in a myriad of different ways. By praying and looking and accepting yourself, you can find the steps that you enjoy.

Not everyone likes to run. If you don't, that's OK; it's not a requirement for good health. Think of the last chapter's **(A)—Accept yourself.** You're not defective if you don't like to run. You're not going to fail to meet your goals if you're not out there running twenty miles every week. The beauty of this body God designed for you is that it responds very well to everyday, moderate physical exercise.

This leads us nicely into the **(B)—Be physically active.** Does it mean you have to go out tomorrow and run twenty miles? No. Does it mean you need to find ways in your daily life to increase your physical activity? Yes. *You cannot achieve the health benefits you desire without physical activity and exercise.* Remember, God designed your body to be physically active. In this chapter, you've read some of the benefits He's preloaded into your design. And the beauty about God is that the more you study about this body He gave you in relation to physical exercise, the more benefits you'll learn. We've all learned so much over the past twenty years, and there's more to discover and celebrate.

Please also know that it's not too late—once a couch potato, not always a couch potato. You are not destined to grow roots out of your eyes. Just get up off that couch and move around. One of the most heartening areas of research shows the benefits of physical exercise for those who were sedentary. According to the American Heart Association's "Statement on Exercise: Benefits and Recommendations for Physical Activity Programs for All Americans," "The greatest potential for reduced mortality is in the sedentary who become moderately active."[1] If you get up off the couch, you will reap incredible health benefits, and doing it doesn't involve running a marathon!

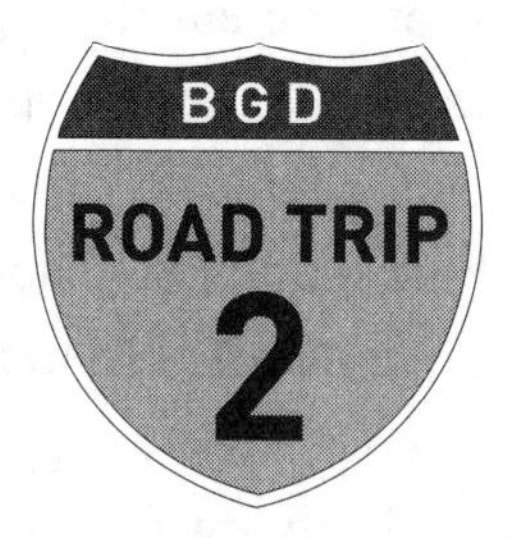

This seems like an excellent time for a road trip, metaphorically speaking. I want you to go back through your list of rooms and think about how you can increase the number of steps you take during the day. What are the ways, right now, you can start to be more active? Here are a couple you might think of, but by no means limit yourself to my limited imagination. Outdo me in creativity!

- Walk more places. This is a pretty simple addition since most of us are already walking as a part of our day. Stop thinking about the amount of distance you walk as a negative and begin to look at those steps as a positive way to get closer to the body God designed for you. Park farther away from work or the shopping mall and walk the extra distance. Take a walk during your break or lunchtime. Several times during your day, walk to talk to a co-worker instead of using the phone. ("Yes, but what about productivity?" you say. "Isn't it more productive to call?" Actually, by getting up and moving around, you can increase your productivity by taking that physical break. The body God designed was simply not meant to sit in a cubicle for eight hours straight, moving inches at best, and do its best work. Your body and mind need the increased circulation and the relief from repetitive motion through physical movement to function better. So, it's OK. You'll be more productive if you occasionally get up and move around.)

- Play more. When was the last time you got out and threw a ball or engaged in some sort of sport? How about getting out with your kids or your dog and just running around? Family interaction was not meant to only take place within the confines of four walls. Your kids are only young once. It's not a waste of time or an imposition on your time to spend time with them. And when your children merely accompany you on your errands, being carted along doing what you have to do, that's not really what I'm talking about here. Get out and play with your kids, going where they want to go and doing what they want to do—and make it something you do outside as much as possible. That's why coats, hats, and gloves were invented, for those of us in chillier climates. Don't have kids? What about your spouse, significant other, or a friend?

- Be vigorous in your chores. Remember the example earlier of piling everything on the bottom of the stairs so you only had to make one trip? That might be efficient, but it does nothing toward increasing your physical activity. Go up and down the stairs multiple times. Do your chores more quickly and energetically. "Oh, come on!" you may be saying to yourself. "Housework? Good for you?" Actually, it appears to be true. A study called "Physical Activity and Breast Cancer Risk: The European Prospective Investigation Into Cancer and Nutrition," published in the December 2006 edition of *Cancer Epidemiology, Biomarkers & Prevention* (is that scholarly enough for you?), found that regular housework reduced breast cancer risks in women because of its physical activity benefits.[2] Think of it this way: you, like many people, may dislike housework. But now there's a really great reason to do it. Even though this study used two hundred thousand European women, I would venture to guess that American women—and men—can benefit from rigorous household chores as well.

- Get outside and tend that garden. One of the activities often cited as physically beneficial is getting out and working in your yard. All that bending, stretching, lifting, and moving around is actually a miniworkout—with weeds. (Have you ever seen a seriously overweight landscaper? I doubt it.) Sure, you can get someone else to do it for you, but you may want to rethink hiring this out, especially if you're having difficulty coming up with other ways to increase your physical activity. Gardening and yard work are both a physical and a creative enterprise. They are athletic and aesthetic. They are also what all of us were originally designed for, if you go back far enough.

In going online and doing research for this chapter, I came across a couple of acrostics that I really like, so I'll pass them along to you as you consider how you can **(B)—Be physically active**. The first comes from the American Heart Association in its guidelines for choosing physical activity. They call it the F-I-T formula.[3] *F* stands for frequency, *I* stands for intensity, and *T* stands for time. The higher each category is, the quicker you can achieve fitness. Here's how the F-I-T formula works: Say you start by walking around your neighborhood. You start out with the *F*, or frequency, at three times a week. Under the *I* for intensity, you're going to go a mile, and your *T* for time is thirty minutes. This level of F-I-T is going to provide a certain level of health benefit and for many people is a realistic place to start. In order to increase in fitness, you increase each of the components over time. For frequency, you work to where you can go five times a week at a twenty-minute-mile pace for forty minutes. You've increased the F-I-T and your fitness. You may decide to shoot for the moon and work toward five times a week jogging a ten-minute-mile pace for forty minutes. Welcome to the club! There's your twenty miles a week. To make it possible for people to stick with a program, the American Heart Association (AHA) recommends thirty minutes of moderate to vigorous exercise on most days for those who are able. This can be thirty minutes in one shot, or it can be broken up into smaller chunks. You may start by taking a single ten-minute walk during the day and work up in frequency to twice a day or add more time during each of the walks. There are many ways to get that thirty minutes a day. There's wisdom in finding several ways that make sense for your schedule and circumstances. (Though, remember, doing nothing doesn't make sense.)

As a caveat here, the AHA recommends that you check in with your doctor before starting any type of vigorous exercise program. If you have a health condition that makes certain activities harmful, you'll also want to see your doctor. If you start off too quickly or too hard, you may end up exhausted, injured, and dispirited. Remember, slow and steady wins the race. Your body is being transformed by the renewing of your physical strength and stamina. This is a process and a journey, and God will be with you.

The other acrostic I really like came from a British health insurance Web site! (That's the power and joy of the Internet, I guess.) The site used the acrostic S-M-A-R-T for how to stay motivated when beginning an exercise program.[4] S-M-A-R-T helps you remember that your activity should be:

- S—Specific. You already know your destination; you simply have to figure out where you're going to place your first step, and your second, and then the one after that. Be specific in what you're going to do tomorrow to increase your physical activity. It doesn't have to be thirty things. Start out with one and then do it.

- M—Measurable. Instead of saying, "I'm going to walk farther each day," say to yourself, "I'm going to park three blocks away from my workplace and walk both to and from work each day." Or you could say, "I'm going to walk twice around my block Monday through Friday. On the weekends, I'm going to walk that distance twice a day." That's both specific and measurable.
- A—Achievable. You're a recovering couch potato, and you say to yourself, "It's January, and I'm going to run a marathon by June." This is not achievable. However, with the proper training and time, you could run a 10K race. If your goals are not achievable you won't, by definition, achieve them. You will fail, become discouraged, and probably give up. This is not a recipe for success. However, if you grasp the concept of baby steps and make your goals achievable, you'll succeed. Success breeds more success. Remember, each baby step achieved, though small, adds up to miles.
- R—Realistic. This is akin to achievable. Please make your goals realistic for you, not for who you want to be or think you should be or the person next door. Make goals that are realistic for you right now. Remember the **(A)—Accept yourself** as you are working toward the **(B)—Be physically active**. It's OK to start small. When you're successful, you'll be ready to move on that much more quickly. Surprise yourself!

- T—Time based. It's OK to allot yourself time to be more physically active. This is not a waste of time but a fulfillment of it. If it usually takes you three hours to clean the house, set yourself a goal to do it more quickly and get it done in two. If you start out taking forty minutes to walk a mile, set yourself a goal to shave off a couple of minutes each week.

Again, be creative. Pray and ask God to alert you to ways you can naturally increase your physical activity each day. Then take advantage of them. Begin to see yourself as an active person, not a sedentary one. Be invested and involved in each moment. Think of yourself as a physical person. This is who God created you to be and the body He made for you. Your body truly was designed by God, and physical activity is an important step to reclaiming it.

Personal Activity Plan

Please don't groan at this heading. You need a plan. Why? Because not having a plan has been pretty ineffective for you, right? OK, so it's time to try actually *planning* how you're going to be more active. Then, once you have your plan in place, you'll have a F-I-T and S-M-A-R-T direction to take.

As you've been reading this chapter, hopefully you have been thinking to yourself, "I could do that," regarding increasing your physical activity each day. After all, we're not talking about training for the Boston Marathon next month. Rather, we're talking about baby steps to fitness. I'm not here to dictate to you what those baby steps are. I don't know you and your lifestyle, where you live and work, or how much physical activity you're getting now. What I do know is that if you're like most adults, you don't get enough physical activity in your day and you feel *really lousy* about it. It's time to stop feeling lousy and start feeling good—good about yourself and good about the baby steps you're going to outline as a way to increase your fitness level.

Let's start small. I want you to identify and write down three small ways you're going to increase your physical activity each day. We're going to call this your Personal Activity Plan. Get a small spiral-bound notebook that can go into your glove box, work drawer, or purse. Write down your goals and what you've accomplished. Keep it with you in a convenient place as an accountability tool, a reminder of your reasons for striving to reclaim the body God designed for you.

Make a heading for each day—one page per day—because your days are not all the same. If you work a traditional Monday-through-Friday schedule, that means you actually have a weekend when you may have greater flexibility to increase your physical activity. However, please remember two words of caution: *weekend warrior.* You do not want to become a weekend warrior who does virtually nothing physical all week long and then attempts to relive the glory days of youth on Saturday and Sunday. Weekend warriors end up in emergency rooms. The goal here is not to save up all your weekly physical activity to expend in a frenzy over the weekend. Instead, the goal is to make physical activity a part of every day. If you're able to get in some extended, appropriate exercise on those days when you have more discretionary time, that's wonderful, but fitness is a seven-day-a-week proposition.

Again, start small. Maybe it's taking the stairs at work instead of the elevator. Maybe it's parking in an outer lot and walking in. Maybe it's taking the dog for a walk in the morning instead of just letting Rover outside. Maybe it's paying attention to the pace of your work at home and doing it with more energy and speed. If you're already doing some level of physical activity, make a plan to incrementally increase that activity.

Be specific. Think of something you can measure: amounts of time, distances, and so forth. This will help give you parameters and a goal to reach. Be realistic. Success breeds success. The ways you choose need to be something you can actually accomplish each day. Do you remember the biblical admonition, "Fathers, do not exasperate your children, so that they will not lose heart" (Colossians 3:21, NASU)? If you exasperate yourself by unrealistic, out-of-proportion planning, you'll lose heart and quit. If you start out a little "too small," you'll amaze yourself and feel much better about what you're able to do. Once you begin to work on this day by day, your fitness level will increase, and you can make informed changes to your goals.

For your Personal Activity Plan, mark down the ways in which you are increasing your level of physical activity each day. Use the day before to help you make decisions about the next day. You want to build daily on your successes. Because we are such creatures of habit, look for activities during each day of the week that can be replicated. For example, if you can park farther away at work or take the stairs to your floor instead of the elevator or escalator, plan to make a habit of these changes. Once they are a habit, you can add others and progressively increase your activity level. These are lifestyle changes you're making, and the more you can ingrain them as habits and daily patterns, the less you'll have to think about them and the more quickly they'll just be part of your normal routine.

If it's been awhile since physical activity was normal for you, realize this will probably feel a little abnormal. You may feel a little strange parking three hundred yards from your work and leaving your car in the next building's parking lot. If people look at you askew and ask what in the world you're doing that for, just explain you're trying to get a little more exercise each day. Trust me; they'll nod their heads in agreement. It won't seem strange to them; it will seem *admirable*.

Until this becomes a habit, look over your activity plan each day in the morning. This will help you to be in that mental mode at the start of your day. It's going to take awhile for your brain to shift from the time-is-money-is-convenience mode to the my-health-is-worth-the-time mode. Focus at the start of your day on what you want to accomplish physically that day and you'll be more apt to avoid the old, sedentary habits.

I know this may seem pedestrian (that's a pun, for all you walkers out there), but I also want you to mark off each activity completed daily. There should be checkmarks and stars and exclamation points all over your Personal Activity Plan. You must be your own best cheerleader on this. Don't sit around waiting for someone else to do it for you. I've told you what to do, but you have to live it each day. Any real success you have will be yours to accomplish and yours to celebrate.

Start celebrating today!

Above all, please remember that what you're working toward is what God intended for you in the first place. He placed us in a garden and gave us physical activity to accomplish. Our bodies were made for this.

Father, I praise You for the body You've given me. Help me to devote myself to health by making each day a physically active one. Allow me to know the blessings You have built into a physically active body. Guard me from becoming discouraged. Give me wisdom to see how I can be more physically active each day. Amen.

Chapter 3

Doughnuts: The New Forbidden Fruit

When the woman saw that the fruit of the tree was good for food and pleasing to the eye, and also desirable for gaining wisdom, she took some and ate it. She also gave some to her husband, who was with her, and he ate it.

—Genesis 3:6

Why, you may wonder, are we still in Genesis? The whole "physical activity" chapter started off with Genesis 2:8 and we have made it only to Genesis 3:6. Talk about baby steps!

There are many valuable lessons to be found in the story of Adam and Eve in the garden. One of them is the concept that not everything that tastes good is good for you. Learning that lesson has ended up being one of our fundamental problems. So let's add it to the idea of fitness from chapter 2 and say, "Fitness and food are fundamentals for a body God designed." Fitness and food are fundamental, which means I'm covering them first, before you progress into more nuanced barriers to health and fitness. You're still in the "genesis," if you will, of discovering what you need to know about your body that God designed, so have patience and keep reading!

So far you've taken the baby steps of **(A)—Accept yourself** and **(B)—Be physically active**. Those are great, in and of themselves, but they're simply not enough. It's also imperative that you and I learn to **(C)—Choose food wisely**. From the very beginning of time, as it turns out, that's been one of humanity's problems.

Our history with choosing food unwisely started with Eve, the fruit, and the Fall. Now, Eve didn't just grab the fruit and eat it without thinking. Give her some credit. The verse quoted at the beginning of this chapter says Eve had three reasons for eating the fruit: first, she saw it was good for food; second, it was pleasing to the eye; and third, it was desirable for gaining wisdom. These are pretty good reasons, and I can almost hear her convincing herself that eating the fruit was really a good thing. I don't think she was deliberately trying to disobey God. I don't think it had gone that far. It was all about the fruit—the perceived benefits of her actions—and not the consequences. I can completely understand her thinking on this. After all, I do it myself.

Bear with me as we look at the chronology of the forbidden fruit for just a minute because it will be instructive later on:

- God tells Adam that he can eat of any tree in the garden except one—the tree of the knowledge of good and evil. There's a whole bunch of fruit that's perfectly good and acceptable for him to eat and one kind that isn't. (See Genesis 2:16.)
- In the very next verse, God makes Eve so Adam won't be alone.
- The serpent approaches Eve and sets up the temptation by introducing doubt into God's pronouncement about the forbidden fruit. (See Genesis 3:1.)

- In verse 2, Eve demonstrates that even though she wasn't personally around to hear what God said about fruit, she's aware of the prohibition.
- In verses 3 and 4, the serpent, tempting Eve, calls God's pronouncement into question. Basically, he calls God a liar.
- Eve accepts the lie in verse 5, which brings us to Genesis 3:6, in which Eve eats the forbidden fruit.

This story, of course, is more than just about fruit. God establishes His rules and makes them known to those affected. The serpent calls those rules into question and introduces the temptation to doubt God's Word. Eve and Adam choose to go with doubt and disobey the rules. They immediately feel shame and attempt to hide what they've done. What God intended for them in the garden and in life is now changed because of their disobedience.

How does this work with us today?

For starters, we know that God has established certain truths about our lives and bodies, just as He established the truth about not eating fruit from the tree in the middle of the garden. It's His world, His rules. As He did in the garden, He reveals to us what those rules and their consequences are. Granted, there is no verse that explicitly says, "Thou shalt not eat cupcakes." But there are plenty of verses that speak about living a moderate, self-controlled life and warn against gluttony. God has revealed these truths through Scripture and also through this amazing body He created for each of us. We've known for years what our mothers taught us: to eat all our vegetables, not take too many cookies from the cookie jar, have water and milk instead of soft drinks, and for heaven's sake go outside and play! The more science and research that are done about food and health, the more they illustrate the wisdom of God's plan for moderation and a physically active life. So, as Romans 1:20 says, we're fresh out of excuses.

We also know that the serpent is still around, calling God a liar and trying to compromise our obedience to Him. Satan's desire is not our enlightenment or "freedom" from God's "oppressive" rules and "unfair" consequences. Satan's desire is our destruction and misery. He's not in it for us; he's in it for himself. We believe his lies at our own peril.

Death by Doughnuts

Let's take a look at how this plays out with doughnuts, which I call the new forbidden fruit. I love doughnuts. I could eat a large number of them in one sitting. There's something about the texture of the cake, the sweetness of the icing, the emotional impact of a doughnut, to say nothing of the carbohydrate surge.

For many years, I thought I had doughnuts under control. I could drive past a Dunkin' Donuts and not look twice. I could mosey along past the doughnut case in the grocery store and not feel that twinge of longing. I thought I had doughuts beaten, and then Krispy Kreme came to town. It was an invasion from the South. All of a sudden, everyone was talking about doughnuts. I don't know how it is where you live, but when Krispy Kreme opened its first store in the Seattle area, people waited hours and drove long distances just to get their hands—and mouths—on them. It was a cultural phenomenon. For me, it was a new front in an old battle, an ancient battle that had started with forbidden fruit. Allow me to share the progression that takes place:

- I know that eating too many doughnuts is not good for me or the body God designed for me. I know this because of God's Word and because of the condition of God's creation, my body.

- Even though I know eating too many doughnuts is not good for me, I want to eat more. I am tempted to believe that God's laws apply to everyone else's body but mine. Surely, all those calories, fat, and sugar won't affect me. Surely not. Surely I can eat just one doughnut. Surely not.
- I see that box of Krispy Kreme doughnuts as good for food and pleasing to the eye. (At this point, I veer off from Eve's line of thinking. I couldn't care less about the wisdom part; the first two reasons are good enough for me.)
- Before I know it, I've bought a box and just consumed half a dozen. After all, they're smallish, warm, and soft, and you can eat one in two bites. They take absolutely no time at all to consume.
- As soon as I eat my half-dozen doughnuts, I immediately feel regret and try to hide the truth by folding the box eight times over and stuffing it into the very bottom of the garbage, under last night's onion peels.

This is my Eve moment. By listening to my own desires and believing a lie, I've been tempted right into discrediting a biblical truth from God: not everything that tastes good and looks good is good for you. Or to put it another way, looks can be deceiving. This truth is fundamental and basic. It's one of the premier ways you and I are tempted into choosing food unwisely. If you are going to **(C)—Choose food wisely** and recapture the body God designed for you,

you need to take a look at how you've been deceived into making the wrong food choices.

Deception Has Three *P's*

You may think that *deception* has only one *p* in the middle of the word. Actually, the kind of deception I'm talking about has three *p*'s. They stand for packaging, processing, and portioning. Who is responsible for these three *p*'s? Well, think of the food industry as a little like the serpent in that it is deceptive and does not have your best interests at heart. The company that makes fried pork rinds is not concerned with your cholesterol or blood lipid levels. It's concerned with selling you as many bags of fried pork rinds as it can. (If you don't like fried pork rinds, just substitute any of your favorite empty-calorie snack foods.)

The first *p* of deception—packaging

In order to sell fried pork rinds, the packaging used will highlight any perceived positives and downplay any known negatives. The packaging isn't about delivering information; it's about image. On the packaging, fried pork rinds may be touted as a more nutritious snack than, say, potato chips because fried pork rinds are higher in protein. This, of course, is obvious because potatoes are not made of protein and pork rinds come from the skin of pigs. But image is all about highlighting even the obvious in order to sell the product. Fried pork rinds do have more protein than potato chips, but they are just as high in fat and a lot higher in sodium. The packaging, though, might say "Nutritious Snack" in bold letters and "compared to potato chips" in very, very small letters. Packaging is not merely the vehicle for transporting and storing the food product; packaging is the vehicle to sell it.

Eve thought that something that *looked* good would *be* good, and she fell prey to a misconception that continues to this day. Food packagers are aware of this misconception. So they make every effort to produce packaging that makes food look good. Sometimes, this includes completely obscuring the food itself by covering it up with attractive packaging. The food we can't see is what we're going to eat, covered up by the packaging we can see but can't eat. This makes us buy food for the wrong reason, only because of the way it's packaged.

The second *p* of deception—processing

Food processing used to mean drying strips of meat to make jerky or drying figs and dates so they wouldn't rot. It meant storing fruits and vegetables in a dark, cool hole in the ground so they would last weeks instead of days. This was fairly straightforward processing. People didn't want food to spoil and become inedible. After all, food is perishable.

That was then; this is now. Food processing has become immensely more complicated and confusing. Oh, the goal is still the same—to keep the food from spoiling. The only problem is that the ways the food industry has found to keep it from spoiling aren't always healthy for you. It's a good-news/bad-news kind of scenario. The good news is those cookies in that bag will last for six months in your cupboard (theoretically, of course, since we all know that a bag of cookies is not going to last for six months in anyone's cupboard). The bad news is that in order to last theoretically six months in your cupboard, they are made with hydrogenated oils, which makes them bad for you.

Whenever I think of hydrogenated oils, I think of Crisco. For those of you unfamiliar with this product, it's a large round container of, essentially, solid fat. Introduced to the world in 1911, Crisco was an amazing product. You could cook with it, fry with it, and bake with it. In 1923, it was put in an airtight can, making it even more amazing, with a shelf life of two years unopened and a year if opened. Imagine the progress of a product that could last up to a year, even if opened, in 1923![1]

The amazing longevity of Crisco had to do with the processing of the oil. The process was called hydrogenation. The chemical makeup of oil, vegetable oil in this case, was altered through the introduction of hydrogen. This produced a stable, solid fat compound, which allowed for a great leap forward in shelf life. It had only one major drawback that was not discovered until years later. It turns out that the hydrogenation process produces a bad type of fat called trans fatty acids or trans fat. Trans fats have been shown to increase your ratio of bad cholesterol and contribute to coronary heart disease.[2] You've now become acquainted with what is often called the law of unintended consequences. What started out as a good thing—food that didn't spoil—ended up as a bad thing—food that can clog your arteries.

As a side note, I went to www.crisco.com (yes, Crisco has its own Web site) and was pleased to find out that it's been reformulated as of 2007, and now a serving of Crisco has zero trans fats. Of course, there's snazzy packaging to herald this important new truth.

Food processing has also produced another unintended consequence. Food processing has allowed us to obtain whatever type of food we want without having to bother to make it ourselves. Food processing has allowed us to merge food with convenience. Now, we have convenience food, also known as snack food, junk food, munchies, or goodies. Without a great deal of time or effort, we are able to eat pretty much what we want. And what we seem to want are cookies, crackers, snack food, junk food of all sorts.

All of this processed food is generally high in calories, sugar, fat, and often sodium. Let's take a look at the flour used in making a variety of snacks. The flour used in baking these goodies is usually highly processed. It is generally referred to as white or processed flour. With white flour, components of the grain fiber are removed to make it lighter, which—and here's one of its values to the food industry—

makes it require less flour to make products. Because it's lighter, air pockets form more easily during proofing so the dough rises higher and makes the loaf look bigger. Instead of buying bread, you're buying air, which works out great for the manufacturers because air doesn't cost *them* anything. If they used whole-wheat flour, why, they'd have to use more flour to achieve the same loaf dimension, and it would cost more to ship because it would weigh more.

Are you getting the idea here that there's a lot more that goes into the processing of your food than what's going to be the best food for you?

Allow me to share one more unintended consequence of white, processed flour. Because much of the fiber has been milled out, it's much easier for your body to convert the carbohydrates in the flour into sugar. In fact, these products can hit your bloodstream like gangbusters. No need for them to mull around in your gut for an hour or two, digesting through the bran and the endosperm of the wheat. Oh no, they're on the fast track into your bloodstream. It's in a form that your body can use right now, whether or not your body is ready to accept the flood.

Let's back up for a minute and go over the three basic components of your food: proteins, fats, and carbohydrates.

- Proteins are meats, poultry, dairy, legumes (beans).
- Fats? Well, I'll explain the complexities of fats in a later chapter.
- Carbohydrates are grains, vegetables, and fruits.

For right now, let's concentrate on the carbohydrate side of things. There are complex carbohydrates and simple carbohydrates. Sugar is a simple carbohydrate made from plants. Sugar is in such a simple form that the body can suck it up in no time. The digestion of simple sugars is pretty quick; sugar hits your bloodstream with a bang.

Sugar in the bloodstream is called glucose. Through research into diabetes, the word *glycemic*, which derives from the word *glucose*, has been invented to indicate how different types of food are digested and deliver their glucose punch. The scale that was developed for rating these different foods is called the "glycemic index." The fast-and-furious rate at which these foods are translated into sugar by the body is called "glycemic load."

"Glycemic index" and "glycemic load"—where did all this come from? This concept was introduced to the United States in 1999 through a book by Jennie Brand-Miller, PhD, called *The Glucose Revolution: The Authoritative Guide to the Glycemic Index*. It was first published under a different name in Australia, and the University of Sydney has a Web site devoted to the glycemic index (GI) of foods. It contains the latest GI data and resources. Log on to www.glycemicindex.com, and you'll find a search engine where you can type in a type of food, such as "fruit," and you'll get ninety different types of fruit with each one's glycemic index and glycemic load. You can also go to www.calvin.biochem.usyd.edu.au/GIBD to find information about specific foods.

So, just what is the glycemic index? Here is the definition from the University of Sydney Web site: "The glycemic index is a ranking of carbohydrates on a scale of 0 to 100 according to the extent to which they raise blood sugar levels after eating. Foods with a high GI are those which are rapidly digested and absorbed and result in marked fluctuations in blood sugar levels. Low GI foods, by virtue of their slow digestion and absorption, produce gradual rises in blood sugar and insulin levels and have proven benefits for health."[3] At www.glycemicindex.com, you can download an American Diabetes Association 2006 *Practical Use of the GI* by Johanna Burani, MS, RD, CDE.

Since 1999, the glycemic index has been modified to include the idea of glycemic load. Glycemic load was developed because the glycemic index doesn't tell you how many carbohydrates are in a serving. The classic example comes from the lowly carrot. On the GI, carrots have a rating of 131, compared to 100 for white bread and 92 for table sugar. Common sense dictates that, surely, eating carrots is better for you than eating table sugar.

Here's where the problem comes in: the GI is based on how quickly the body will turn 50 grams of a particular food's carbohydrates into sugar. But a serving of carrots has only 4 grams of carbohydrates. In other words, you'd need to eat a pound and a half of carrots to eat 50 grams! So the GL (glycemic load) takes the GI of a food and multiplies it by the number of carbohydrates in a serving. In the carrot example, it would be 1.31 (131 percent) x 4 = 5.24, thereby reducing its glycemic index rating under glycemic load.

If all of this makes you feel like you've gone back to middle school math, relax. The shortened version is to be aware of the impact on your blood sugar levels of highly processed foods and avoid foods that rank highest on the GI.

If you repeatedly eat foods that are high on the glycemic index, it's the equivalent of jump-starting your body over and over with high bursts of blood sugar. Over time, you can develop a condition known as insulin resistance, which contributes to the onset of type 2 diabetes. (Type 2 diabetes is the type that derives from your lifestyle and not your genetics, and it is seriously on the rise in this country.) Again, here are unintended consequences.

What this means in real life is that it's not just those doughnuts that can give you problems. It's also all those snacks made with highly processed white flour. Processing brings us convenience to be sure, but convenience brings along uninvited houseguests that take up residence in your bloodstream and coronary arteries. What looks and tastes good isn't always good for you.

The third *p* of deception—portioning

Just a word about portioning before we go on a BGD Road Trip. This used to be one of the food industry's best-kept little secrets. Portioning works in two ways when it comes to food. The first way is the oversized portion, usually provided at restaurants, fast-food outlets, and your Aunt Minnie's house at Thanksgiving. This is the pumped-up-on-steroids portion. It's the fourth of pie that masquerades as "one slice." It's the two cups of mashed potatoes and gravy that parade as a "single helping," allowing you to go back for seconds when the first was really first, second, and third helpings all rolled into one. It's the salad-plate-sized cookie that only counts as "one cookie."

The second deception when it comes to portioning is the itsy, bitsy portion, usually hidden away on—you guessed it—food packaging. It's finding out by reading the fine print that the salad-plate-sized cookie really represents four servings at 150 calories a piece. Do you remember that bag of cookies in the pantry that's supposed to last six months but never does? It's because when you want some cookies, you go in and grab three or four or more. That's a serving, right? Wrong. If you'll get out your magnifying glass, you'll see that a single cookie is a serving. By grabbing a handful, you've just eaten five servings, not one.

The people who put the cookies in that bag are catching on to the trend to count calories. The smaller they can make the "portion," the fewer calories they have to list on the package. They can say, "Just 50 calories per serving!" Of course, normal people will eat four servings without even blinking and still reach in for more. Be warned. Watch both the calories and the serving size. Only by adding them together can you get past this deception and on to the truth of what you're actually consuming.

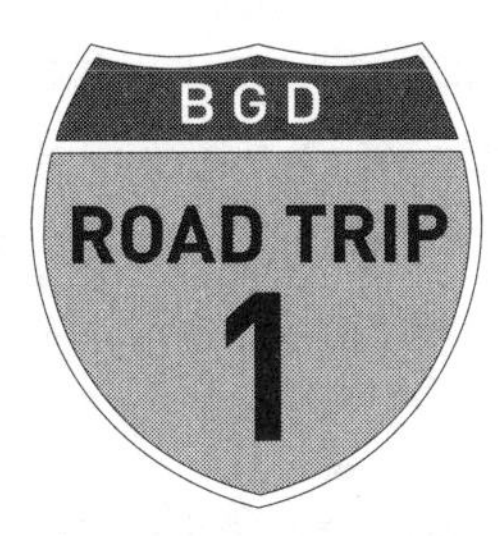

Once again, please put down this book and pick up a notebook. You're going on a journey to your kitchen. I want you to go through your cupboards, drawers, and cabinets. Pull out all those boxes, bags, or containers of packaged, processed foods. Put on your Sherlock Holmes hat and start investigating just what is in those cookies you've been scarfing down after dinner without really thinking as you're watching television, not to mention that bag of chips or fried pork rinds. Go for the items you eat as snack food or comfort food, instead of "real food" like vegetables and protein. (Of course, if packaged convenience food constitutes your "real food," I think you already sense the need for some change in the air.)

Write down each item. Make columns for portion size, calories per serving, trans fat grams, total fat grams (write this down now, and we'll come back later to use it), sugar grams, and sodium grams. Take out the packages one at a time and fill in the columns.

Just for fun, figure out the following:

- How many total calories does all this food represent?
- If one pound of body fat comes from 3,500 calories, how many pounds does this food represent?

- How long, realistically, would it take you to eat all this food? Do you have to replenish your stash every couple of days? Once a week? How many calories per day of this food are you really going through?
- How much fat are you getting through this food? How many grams of trans fats does this food represent?
- How about the portion size? Did it surprise you to know that a single cookie is considered a serving?
- How does your definition of a "serving" measure up to what the packaging says is a "serving"?
- How many of their servings does your serving represent?

You've probably just been struck with a cold wave of reality. All of those attractive, tasty snacks and treats that seem so harmless individually can sure add up. And where they're adding up is around your middle and on your bathroom scale. It's time to recognize the truth of the food you choose to eat and make a decision to **(C)—Choose food wisely**.

The Whole Truth

I have a name for the packaged, processed foods we've been talking about—I call them "fragmented foods." They look like the real deal, but important elements have been eliminated, scrubbed off, and processed out. They are high in calories but low in nutrition. They tempt us with their ready accessibility. Even though they are a *fragment* of what we really need, they are becoming the *whole* of our choices. It's time to return to whole foods as nutrition.

By *whole foods* I mean foods that are complete in and of themselves. Take an apple, for instance, or any fruit or vegetable. A fruit or vegetable is the ultimate convenience food. You pick one up and eat it. All you need to do is wash it. You don't need to process it. God designed fruits and vegetables to be nutritious inside and out. The rind or skin is often packed full of important nutrients, to say nothing of fiber. Protein is also a whole food. A serving of meat, fish, or poultry is complete in itself. You season it and cook it, but you don't have to process it or alter it chemically.

Another benefit of whole foods is the fiber they provide. Our bodies need fiber to keep foods moving through our digestive and alimentary systems. Our intestines and colon need fiber to operate efficiently. Fiber also takes longer to digest, which means the nutrients and calories in the fiber are delivered to the bloodstream more slowly over time. Our blood sugar levels don't spike up so rapidly that they require our pancreas to counter by increasing amounts of insulin into our bloodstream. Fiber keeps our systems from having to be so reactive; they can respond to the foods we eat instead of having to react to massive dumps of calories, sugars, and sodium.

In real life, this means we should be reaching more into the produce drawer in our refrigerator than the snack shelf in our cupboard or pantry. How is your cupboard doing compared to your produce bin? Just as you needed to go into your closet and accept the truth about your size, you need to go into your kitchen and accept the truth of what you eat. Just because something is called a "snack" food doesn't mean that it's being eaten just as a snack. For too many of us, this category of food takes up a significant portion of our daily and weekly food choices. Six doughnuts isn't a snack; six doughnuts is a meal. It's the same for you as it is for me.

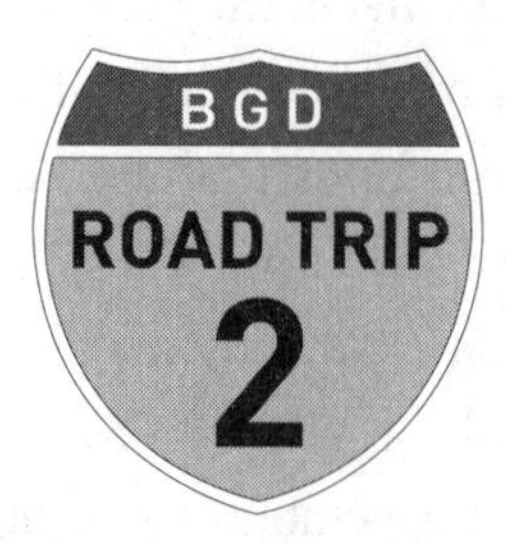

It's impossible for me to tell you just what to eat each day, but I can give you guidelines and knowledge and help you figure it out for yourself. Frankly, I venture to guess that most of you already have a pretty good working knowledge of many things you should avoid just by watching television or picking up a newspaper. You've probably seen the "healthy tips" banner scroll across the homepage of your Internet Service Provider. More and more (and by that I mean as more and more of us age), health information is available. The trick is taking the available information and making it personally practical. That's where Road Trip #2 comes in.

Now, Road Trip #1 in this chapter was probably pretty depressing. After all, you had to go into your kitchen and pull out all your happy comfort food—only to find it wasn't so happy and comforting for your health. (If you really want to be masochistic, don't stop at the kitchen. Do the same thing with all your other "hiding places," you know, where you keep your hidden caches of food. It could be your desk at the office, in your car, in the back of your sock drawer—wherever you've got it, pull it out. Add *that* to your kitchen totals.)

Yes, the last road trip might have seemed like a summer car ride to Uncle Ernie's in the family station wagon—endless and unpleasant. It was necessary, however, for you to come face-to-face with one of food's fundamentals. If it goes in your mouth, it counts. Snack and convenience foods, by their very throwaway nature, can delude us into thinking that their calories don't really count. They do count, and they also count up.

Snack and convenience foods are often directly responsible for our excess weight. We eat them mindlessly, thoughtlessly, mechanically, as an accompaniment to some other activity, such as reading or watching television. In one of life's little ironies, we seldom actually eat veggies when we're "vegging."

Even though snack foods are rarely eaten during an official meal, their calories and content still count, and they definitely affect our health. One of the best things you can do is give up snacking. Eat only at mealtime. If you get a little hungry, drink some water or get up and move around to distract yourself. Being a little hungry is fine. It doesn't hurt you. It may seem uncomfortable at first, but it's a feeling that will go away on its own. Wait to eat until you experience real hunger, then sit down and have a well-balanced meal. Or, if you insist upon having a midmorning or late-afternoon snack, make it a piece of fruit or some cut-up vegetables.

For this happier road trip, I want you to head out on the road called the Information Superhighway, also known as the Internet. It'll be easier if you have a computer at home, but if you don't, yours will be a true road trip down to a friend or relative's house or to your local library. I want you to go onto a great Web site that will help you to **(C)—Choose food wisely**. It's found at www.MyPyramid.gov.

This is the Web site that gives information on the federal government's food pyramid. The food pyramid is a dietary guideline for all ages and activity levels. You can even customize your own pyramid based on your age, weight, sex, level of physical activity, and whether or not you want to maintain or lose weight. It's free, it's fun (lots of graphics and bright colors), and it's fairly easy to use. The amount of information you can read through and print up is voluminous and helpful. You can get a personalized plan that shows you not only how much of each food group to eat daily but also gives you suggestions and choices. Give yourself at least thirty minutes to peruse the site. It's point-and-click easy. Provided by the U.S. Department of Agriculture (USDA), you paid for it with your tax dollars, so you might as well take advantage of it.

When you're on the homepage on www.MyPyramid.gov, look in the upper right-hand corner where it says "My Pyramid Plan." Put in your age, sex, weight (optional but I highly recommend you be honest and put yours in), and daily activity level (not your desired or hoped for or anticipated activity level but what you really do every day). Got your answers in? Hit "Submit."

The site will create a personal pyramid for you to use as a dietary guideline. On the right-hand side of the screen, you can see your plan, and you can print a copy for yourself. You can also obtain a "meal-tracking worksheet" that you can print out to use daily.

Go ahead and print out your meal-tracking worksheet. Your reaction to the information it contains will probably be similar to mine. It can come as a surprise to see how many fruits and vegetables we're supposed to eat and how little of fats and sugars. Our challenge is that our highly processed packaged foods are generally the exact opposite of what we're supposed to be eating—they have little or no fruits and vegetables and lots of fats and sugars. This is the challenge of **(C)—Choose**

food wisely. What we're *used* to eating isn't what we *should* be eating. It will mean making intentional changes to our food choices.

Put your copy of your meal-tracking worksheet in your kitchen. Put it wherever most of your snack and convenience foods are kept: your freezer door (if you go for ice cream and processed frozen dinners) or your cabinet door (if you go for bags of chips and boxes of crackers and cookies). I don't expect you to start using the worksheet tomorrow. That would be great, but I don't expect it. You probably shouldn't place that expectation on yourself either. For now, this is just to remind you about the kinds of choices you will need to make to achieve the body God designed for you.

Some of you may think it's strange to use something generated by the government to gain understanding into biblical principles. However, the knowledge and insight gained through a study of God's creation (the human body) has contributed to a plan of eating that is tailored to a body's best interests and health. Secular science and research uncover the wisdom and knowledge that were placed in creation by our loving Father. I'm not saying the government is divine or that the plan is inspired, but I am saying that this plan is based on knowledge about the body God has created. I do believe it will help you down the road to your goals.

Start looking over your personal pyramid and memorize the guidelines involved. Get to know how many servings of the various proteins, grains, dairy, vegetables, and fruits you should be consuming each day as well as your total daily caloric goals. I want you to start using these as templates for analyzing what you're eating. Begin to interrogate yourself about your food choices. Once again, you're gaining knowledge through baby steps. This is a journey, remember?

The Desert of Doughnuts

Does this mean I can never have a doughnut again? No, but it means I shouldn't have six in one sitting. Why? Because it's not good for my body.

God told us we're to love our bodies, not abuse them. In Ephesians, when the apostle Paul speaks of the relationship between husbands and wives, he mentions the love and care we are to have for our bodies almost as a given. He says, "Husbands ought to love their wives as their own bodies. He who loves his wife loves himself. After all, no one ever hated his own body, but he feeds and cares for it, just as Christ does the church" (Ephesians 5:28–29).

What would your spiritual health be like if Christ fed and cared for you spiritually the way you feed and care for yourself physically? If you took Christ's example to heart and fed and cared for yourself physically the way He feeds and cares for you spiritually, what would your physical health be like? The answer to the last question, of course, is you'd be walking around in a body God designed instead of a body designed by packaging, processing, and portions. If you want to have longevity and health, you're going to have to do it God's way. Not much has changed. It was true in the garden, and it's still true today.

Got your meal-tracking worksheet up where you can see it and be reminded? It's not too late to make a positive change in your life. God's on your side, and so am I. Choose truth instead of deception. Eat truthfully and honestly. Watch your sheet and begin to make small, repeatable changes every day—baby steps to victory!

Would all hell break loose if I did eat six doughnuts in one sitting? No, but as I choose food more wisely, my body will become accustomed to proper eating. I'll probably feel a little lousy after eating that many doughnuts as my blood sugar spikes up. And that will help me remember the biblical truth that *not everything that looks good and tastes good is good for me.* Next time I want a doughnut, I may have one, but I won't eat six. There may even come a time when my desire for a doughnut isn't all I think about when I walk into the grocery store or pass that Krispy Kreme store down the street!

> *Father, I need help to choose food wisely. I confess I have chosen the foods I eat for my own reasons. So often my choices were based upon what I wanted and not what my body needed. Help me to look to You for guidance in my food choices. Remind me that my body is Your temple and I must look to You to know how to care for it and feed it. As You guide me in what I should eat today, keep me in Your presence so I can resist the temptation of the evil one. Amen.*

Chapter 4

My Kingdom for Some Chromium

Cursed is the ground because of you; through painful toil you will eat of it all the days of your life. It will produce thorns and thistles for you, and you will eat the plants of the field.

—Genesis 3:17–18

In computerese, there's a phrase, "Garbage in, garbage out," shortened to "GIGO." It means that what you get out of anything is directly related to what you put in. In a simpler day, the phrase would have been "You reapaw what you sow," which is very biblical (Galatians 6:7).

This technological phrase is also completely appropriate in an agrarian setting when it comes to the food we eat. Modern farming and marketing techniques produce a crop that can be lacking in nutrients. We overfarm and leech nutrients from the soil. We use chemicals and pesticides to control weeds and critters. We allow pollutants and toxins in our soil and ground water. We've messed with God's field, and it doesn't always produce as well as it should.

Because of us, the ground truly is cursed. It's taking more and more fertilizers to replenish the soil. It works out to this: depleted nutrients in the soil equal stunted, substandard produce.

The Human Factor

This equation might not be quite as difficult if it weren't for the human factor. If all we needed to do was test the soil, figure out what nutrients are lacking, and make sure to mix the right fertilizer concoction to refortify the soil, that would be fairly simple. Agronomists do it all the time. It's a booming business—companies provide the right concoctions to farmers to make sure their soil is fertile and will support crop production. But, of course, anytime you throw in the human factor, complications arise. (We're still in Genesis, remember?)

In spite of soil depletion, we could get all of the nutrients we need through the food we eat—if we would eat the right food. The problem is we don't. All of us should take to heart the Dietary Guidelines for Americans, which was last updated in 2005 by the U.S. Department of Health and Human Services and the U.S. Department of Agriculture. It's only an eighty-four-page document, and you can obtain it for your reading enjoyment at http://www.health.gov/dietaryguidelines/dga2005/document/pdf/DGA2005.pdf. For those of you with, say, a real life going on, there's a condensed version found on the MyPyramid.gov Web site (http://www.mypyramid.gov/guidelines/index.html). It says:

> The Dietary Guidelines describe a **healthy diet** as one that:
>
> - Emphasizes fruits, vegetables, whole grains, and fat-free or low-fat milk and milk products;
> - Includes lean meats, poultry, fish, beans, eggs, and nuts; and

- Is low in saturated fats, *trans* fats, cholesterol, salt (sodium), and added sugars.

This is pretty much what I talked about in the last chapter. These are all straightforward, commonsense guidelines, so why does the average American have such a problem? *Because we don't actually eat this way.* If we did, most of us would get most of the nutrients we need. But instead, many of us:

- Eat junk food instead of nutritious food.
- Develop eating disorders that rob us of nutritious food.
- Overuse laxatives that leech nutrients from our digestive tracts.
- Take a cornucopia of prescription drugs that compromise our ability to utilize nutrients.
- Overuse alcohol that does the same thing.
- Have messed-up digestive systems that fast-track the nutrients out of our bodies and down the drain.

Whitewashed Food

Let's take a look at the first thing on the list: eating junk food instead of nutritious food. I really don't know who coined the phrase "junk food," but it's an appropriate term. It is, after all, food, in the broad sense of the word, but it is calorie rich and nutrient poor; it's junk, nutritionally speaking. True, it's appealing, tasty, convenient, and satisfying, but it's devoid of what really matters for fueling and equipping the body God designed. Do you remember this reference Jesus made in Matthew 23:27? Speaking of the religious leaders, He said,

"Woe to you, teachers of the law and Pharisees, you hypocrites! You are like whitewashed tombs, which look beautiful on the outside but on the inside are full of dead men's bones and everything unclean."

Junk food is whitewashed tomb food. It looks great on the outside, but there's nothing on the inside but skeletal nutrition and a whole lot of junk. That Twinkie? Whitewashed tomb food. That deep-fried corn dog at the minimart? Whitewashed tomb food. Not nearly so appealing now, is it? Hopefully, having a true picture in your mind of what this stuff really is will help you turn down the siren song of its appeal. When those fried pork rinds start calling your name from the snack aisle, you'll look at the bag, see a heap of dead men's bones inside that very attractive packaging, and start running until you're far, far away.

Yes, run far, far away. Of course, in our current culture, running far, far away from one junk food generally propels you smack into another form of junk food. It's *ubiquitous*, which, according to Merriam-Webster's Online Dictionary, means "existing or being everywhere at the same time; constantly encountered." Isn't that true of junk food? It's everywhere! It's wherever you go! It is possible, however, to be healthy in a nutritional graveyard. You just have to watch where you walk.

In the last chapter, you went to the MyPyramid.gov Web site and printed up your daily meal-tracking worksheet that shows you how many calories are right for you to consume each day and what sort of foods those calories should be derived from. (You did do that, right? If you haven't done it yet, now's the time. Go to page 70 to review the instructions.)

Daily Deposit

OK, you have your meal-tracking worksheets and you're ready to go. Look over the guidelines for food intake. They're not much different from the dietary guidelines above, are they? There's a reason. The bulk of your calories should be from fruits, vegetables, whole grains, low-fat milk products, lean meats, etc. These foods actually contain the nutrients your body needs to function properly. Put another way, it's as if you have a certain number of calories per day in the "bank." With that amount, you will "purchase" or make your food choices. Your goal is twofold: (1) You don't want to spend more calories than you have in your bank. There are no rewards for opening up a bigger account. A bigger account means you're a bigger size. (2) You want to invest your calories in the right mix of nutrients in order to enjoy a health dividend.

My pyramid says I have 2,400 daily calories a day in the "bank," figured for my gender, age, and activity level. Here's how I could be spending that on any given day:

- In the morning, too late getting out the door for breakfast, I make a Starbucks run and get a venti café mocha with whipped cream. Of course, I compromise and choose nonfat milk in the mocha. I've just made a withdrawal of 390 calories. But a mocha's not really breakfast because it's a drink, so it doesn't count as food. For food, I order a blueberry scone and withdraw another 480 calories. I have a 2,400 calorie balance for the day, and I've just deducted 870 calories, or 36.25 percent, of my daily total. (How do I know the calories in these items? Why, Starbucks is happy to share what it calls its nutrition information at http://www.starbucks.com/retail/nutrition_info.asp?cookie%5Ftest=1. You can look up either beverages or food. Put in your zip code and you can even pull up the shop you frequent and get detailed nutrition information about all its locally produced baked goods. Just a note of caution—they're a bit of an eye opener.)

- For lunch, I head out to McDonald's for a quick bite because I'm pressed for time. I'm mindful of breakfast, so I get a classic grilled chicken sandwich (420 calories) and a small order of fries (250 calories)—all things in moderation. Top that off with a carton of low-fat milk (100 calories) and lunch is now responsible for 770 calories of my 2,400 per day, or 32 percent.
- At the end of a long day, it's home for dinner and vegetable lasagna! Now, the package says the serving size is one cup, but that's not nearly enough. So it's 2 cups of vegetable lasagna (because veggie lasagna is certainly better than, say, Italian sausage lasagna) at 440 calories. Next, a multigrain English muffin with butter at 200 calories, a small green salad with dressing at 170 calories, and a glass of water. That's 810 calories of my 2,400, or 33.75 percent.

All told, I've eaten 2,450 calories, pretty close to my daily total. What's 50 calories here or there among friends? Of course, I didn't factor in the candy bar in the afternoon (250 calories) or the ice cream I had after dinner (350 calories), but who's counting? Oh, yeah, we are. I've now eaten 650 calories more than my daily guidelines tell me, or about 25 percent more calories than I should have had for the day.

Oh, I failed to mention that in order to have this level of caloric intake, I'm supposed to get in at least thirty to sixty minutes of physical exercise each day. It was kind of busy today, and I really did *mean* to get out and jog before work, but it just didn't happen. So, actually,

I really should deduct 200 calories, according to my tracking sheet, which means I'm now at 850 calories over for the day.

And what about the food choices on my worksheet? Well, I've probably had the right amount of grains, but at least half of them should have been whole wheat, and I didn't really get anywhere near that. My vegetables came from the lettuce leaf and tomato on the chicken sandwich, the cooked veggies in the veggie lasagna, and the small green salad—maybe three cups, but I doubt it. To be honest, the salad was a couple of baby carrots and some romaine lettuce, so it's hard for me to claim much variety on that one. I ate absolutely no fruit today, except for the blueberries in the blueberry muffin from Starbucks. I got my dairy in the café mocha, the carton of milk at lunch, and the ice cream that I really wasn't going to count unless forced to, but that wasn't nonfat or even low fat. The chicken in the sandwich at lunch counts toward the protein, as well as the cheese in the lasagna, but that wasn't exactly low fat, either.

Are you getting the idea how quickly that bank of daily calories can be taken up by food or beverage items that are calorie rich but nutrient poor? If I only have 2,400 calories per day to fuel my body and give it the vitamins, minerals, and amino acids it requires to perform, I need to do a better job and **(C)—Choose food wisely**.

Let's look at my day and see if we can come up with a different result:

- Instead of hitting the snooze bar three times and then falling back to sleep, I actually get up and jog before going to work. I feel better, and my metabolism is jump-started for the day.
- Instead of hitting Starbucks, I have breakfast at home, consisting of a cup and a half of cooked oatmeal (the slower cooking kind with more of the fiber) at 150

calories with peanut butter thrown in (the protein in the peanut butter helps your breakfast stay in your system and keeps you feeling full longer) at 190 calories. A medium orange at 85 calories and a cup of nonfat milk at 90 calories and my breakfast comes in at 515 calories. That's 355 calories less than the Starbucks run and a lot cheaper.

- Let's say that I still drop by McDonald's for lunch, but instead of choosing the classic grilled chicken sandwich and fries, I choose their Asian salad with grilled chicken at 300 calories with a package of apple slices with caramel dip at 105 calories. Even if I throw in another cup of low-fat milk at 100 calories, I still am only at 505 calories for lunch, 265 calories less than my other trip to McDonald's. Plus, I would have had both fruits and vegetables.
- Now, for dinner, I eat the same thing as before, only, instead of 2 cups of veggie lasagna, I cut that down to a cup and a half. And for the salad, I throw in a couple of broccoli heads and some orange and red pepper strips. My dinner now comes in at around 700 calories.
- I can even substitute a protein bar for the candy bar in the afternoon at 200 calories and low-fat yogurt instead of ice cream at 250 calories. I've made some fairly simple-to-do, real-world changes—no tofu and rice cake meals—and I'm still under my 2,400 day by over 200 calories.

How about my tracking sheet? Well, I've done pretty well with my grains; I chose whole grains with the muffin and the oatmeal. I've eaten several different types of vegetables and had my two cups of fruit. I got my protein from the grilled chicken in the salad, the dairy products I had during the day, and the peanut butter in the morning. I've still had three meals with an afternoon snack and dessert after dinner, and today I consumed almost 900 fewer calories, and I came much closer to my tracking sheet goals.

As a side note, it's amazing to me the way people track all kinds of things, especially if money is involved. I'm thinking of those people who clip coupons and watch sales and save big bucks on their grocery shopping each week. They know what stores to go to for the products they use and when certain sales will be on their favorite items. Their ability to keep track of and maximize their food budget is impressive. Wouldn't it be great if people could be as strategic with their "nutrition budget"?

Overcoming Nutritional Deficits

Junk food and what the food pyramid calls "discretionary calories" use up your nutrient budget without giving much in return. You end up overeating and being undernourished. It's probably the largest reason why we are nutrient deficient.

There are other reasons, however, that I'd just like to touch on. Eating disorders, including anorexia, bulimia, binge eating, and night eating disorder can all play a part in nutrient deficiencies. I see this literally every day in my practice at The Center for Counseling and Health Resources, where we work with clients with eating disorders. When the body and its digestive system are compromised by an eating disorder, it makes it difficult for nutrients, even when consumed, to be properly assimilated and utilized. Some bulimics abuse laxatives, which circumvent the normal gastric processes designed to allow nutrients to flow into the bloodstream during digestion and elimination.

Prescription drugs can interact with other prescription drugs as well as hamper the body's ability to absorb certain nutrients. Add alcohol in the mix, and it can be tough getting the nutrients you need even if you did eat the "right" foods every day.

So, what's the answer? Well, that's been changing recently. It used to be collective wisdom up until a couple of years ago that if you just "ate right," you wouldn't need to take a daily multivitamin. That changed, however, in 2002 when the American Medical Association (AMA) finally admitted what many people already knew; we weren't getting enough of the vitamins and minerals we needed even from a good diet. Because of increasing data from research, the National Academy of Sciences also went about to change the RDAs, or recommended daily amounts, of vitamins and minerals and get them more in line with what was being learned. In an article by Ronald Kotulak in the *Chicago Tribune* on June 19, 2002, this shift in policy on multivitamins by the AMA was explained. It mentioned the now well-known recommendation of five servings of fruits and vegetables per day. But in the article, Dr. Robert Fletcher, who helped write the new AMA guidelines, admitted that even people who ate five servings per day might not get the right amount of certain vitamins for optimal health.[1]

The Magic Pill

So, where does this leave you? Even if you eat a "good" diet, with the recommended five servings of fruits and vegetables per day, you still may not be getting all of the vitamins and minerals you need for optimal health. Since most of us have a hard enough time with the realities of our "nutritional bank," I'm not suggesting that we take on the added computation of trying to calculate how much of which vitamin, mineral, or amino acid is in what we eat. There are other things to do (living life in general comes to mind). As hard as it is just keeping track of the calories and types of food we eat, who wants to add the job of tracking your folic or pantothenic acid or choline or glutamic acid or chromium? Not me, thank you!

I follow the AMA recommendation every day and support my food intake with supplemental vitamins and minerals, and you should, too. Your body cannot make most vitamins (except vitamin D, which requires sunlight) and minerals on its own; you must provide them to your body from an outside source. While eating should still be your primary source of vitamin intake, there's nothing defeatist about taking a good multivitamin and mineral supplement. Look for a multiformula with high bioavailability. In other words, you want a formula that's easy for your body to digest and absorb. Because many of these nutrients are water-soluble, they flush out of your body. This means you need to take them several times over the course of the day in order for a portion of them to be absorbed. What you took in the morning may be down the drain by afternoon.

What this also means is the amount shown on the back of the bottle as the percentage of your daily value (shown often as "%DV") may be several times higher than 100 percent. These daily values were established by the government and calculated to prevent certain nutrient-deficient diseases like scurvy and beriberi. They're a *minimum* requirement and weren't designed to help you attain an optimal level. In addition, each person will absorb and utilize these nutrients at a different rate, depending upon their metabolism, general health, and lifestyle. If you have questions about what multiformula may be right for you, ask your doctor or other health-care professional. Remember, however, that some health-care professionals have just caught up to the 2002 AMA recommendation of a single multivitamin a day and may not totally be on board. Health food stores and supplement chains are also sources of information on the products they sell.

The type of multivitamin we use and sell at the Center has a "serving size" greater than just one pill. Instead, it recommends multiple tablets per day. Taking them in intervals during the day ensures your body has these nutrients available when they're needed. Our Ultra Preventive X formula makes use of the latest research on and expanding knowledge of the role of nutritional supplements in optimal health. (If you want to see how Ultra Preventive X stacks up with other multiformulas, go to our Web site at www.aplaceofhope.com and look for A Place of Hope Store. You can search for this product and see a detailed list of all of the ingredients and percentage of DV.)

In addition, I want to mention two nutritional supplements we've found very helpful for nutritional support. Specifically, they assist in the functioning of the mitochondria. Remember the mitochondria? Think back to high school science. Mitochondria are the engines of the cells. Though tiny, they have a big job to do in the body. Mitochondria in cells act as little furnaces where fat is burned. Mitochondria cannot leave the cells and go to where the fat is, so the fat must come to them. When fat is able to come to them, it can be burned more efficiently and their little engines roar. The body has more energy and less fat. Therein lies the benefit of these two supplements, L-carnitine and coenzyme Q_{10}.

L-carnitine is an amino acid required for the breakdown of fats into energy. It acts as a carrier, transporting fats to the mitochondria, where they can be burned as fuel. The easier fat is burned, the more efficient your physical activity becomes. The more fat burned as fuel, the less stored on your body. The more fat burned, the lower your cholesterol drops. (The L-carnitine formula in use at the Center includes chromium to support healthy glucose metabolism, making it even better for weight loss.)

Coenzyme Q_{10} (ubiquinone) also supports energy production in the mitochondria, revving up your metabolism. In addition, studies have shown it to have antioxidant properties, removing cancer-causing free radicals from your system and functioning as an important cofactor in many enzyme systems, especially in cardiac muscle health.

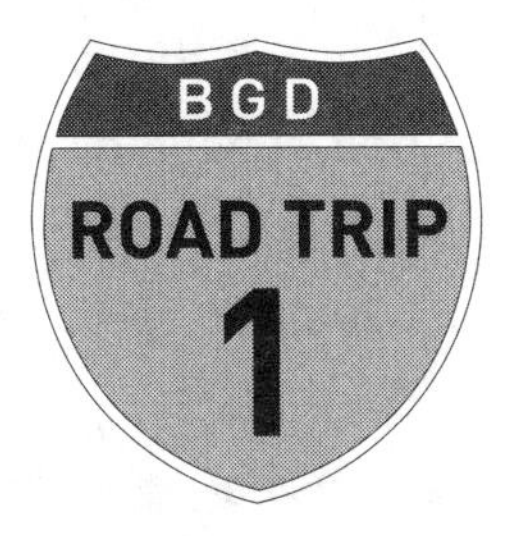

On this road trip, you're going to travel back to your computer. I want you to print up a week's worth of your meal-tracking worksheet. It's been a visual reminder up to this point. Now it's time to start making more direct use of it. I want you to copy or print up a week's worth because I want you to start tracking what you're eating and drinking. If you want to start tomorrow, great. If you want to wait until Monday, that's OK, too, but you need to pick a day to start. Knowledge is power, and you're going to start gaining knowledge about what you eat.

On the tracking sheet you'll see suggestions on the types of grains, vegetables, fruits, milk, meat, and beans to eat. Watch your goals on amounts, and write down everything you eat and drink. Regular sodas, fruit juices, energy drinks, and alcohol all have significant calories that "deduct" from your daily calorie bank, even though they are liquid and not solid. You need to keep track of these items as well.

I also want you to track your caloric intake. This can be a little tricky, but you can do it with preparation. Most food packaging now comes with labels that will give you calories per serving. But remember to watch the serving size. Your definition of a serving of Ben and Jerry's may be vastly different from that on the label. You must follow the label, not your heart, on this.

If you're not sure how many calories or what the serving size is for certain foods, you can get the information in a couple of different ways. You can go online and type in "calorie counting" or something similar in your search box. (A helpful Web site for calorie tracking is www.calorie-count.com.) You can also use those things called *books*. Go to your library or local bookstore and get a book that lists common foods. The advantage of getting your data online is that it's usually updated, but you can still get the general idea from a book and estimate, even if the book doesn't have your specific item. Please don't allow excuses to stop you from tracking your food and caloric intake. It's vital that you work from a platform of truth in order to understand the need to make these changes. Your body deals daily with the "truth" of what you're eating. Now it's time for your mind and heart to catch up and recognize this truth. It's been my experience that keeping track of food and writing down what you eat acts as an accountability tool and helps motivate you to make wiser choices.

Keep track of how you're doing even if you go out to eat. When you go to a restaurant, you can ask for nutrition information about the dishes you choose. For example, I used the Web sites of Starbucks and McDonald's to find out about their offerings. You can check the Web sites of other large restaurant chains you frequent. Otherwise, ask for a brochure. The more you ask, the more these establishments will recognize the need to provide consumers with this information.

You can take your worksheet with you during the day or keep track on a piece of paper and transfer the information later. It is important that you not skip this step. Actually writing down what you eat is a form of knowledge and accountability. Most of us don't pay any attention to what we eat, and then we're surprised that we can't fit into our pants.

Track daily for seven days straight. Watch for patterns. Where do you need to alter your food choices to make sure you're getting the right mix? With the knowledge you gain over a week, I want you to start being proactive and mapping out your food choices for the next day. In order to recapture the body God designed for you, you need to develop strategic thinking. Forewarned is forearmed.

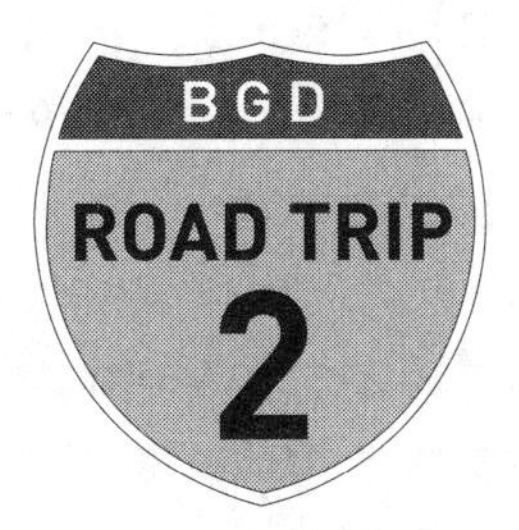

Back-to-back road trips? Yes, because the first is linked to the second. For your second road trip, I want you to investigate nutritional supplements.

If you're not taking a nutritional supplement, I want you to do some research and pick out a good multivitamin formula with high bioavailability. My apologies to the AMA, but if you only have to take it once a day, much of that pill could be gone by lunchtime. Instead, find a formula that let's you take several tablets over the course of the day. Usually, the best time is with a meal.

Some people will react to vitamins taken in the evening, especially those with higher concentrations of B vitamins. These are real energy producers and can cause you to consider it a good idea to vacuum your house at midnight. If they affect you this way, make sure to take them several hours before you go to bed. By all means, use that energy to be productive in the evening, but take them early so you can wind down, relax, and enjoy your rest.

If you're already taking a multivitamin, I want you to get out the bottle and see what sort of percentages each component has. Most should be above the 100 percent range, some significantly so, such as vitamin A, vitamin C, thiamine, riboflavin, niacin, vitamin B_6, folic acid, vitamin B_{12}, pantothenic acid, and magnesium. Vitamin D can be at the 100 percent range because it's the one vitamin your body can produce by itself when you're exposed to sunlight.

The Ultra Preventive X we carry at the Center, made by Douglas Labs (www.douglaslabs.com), also includes a proprietary blend of vegetables, fruits, and herbs formulated into this multivitamin. This can give an added boost to those who find it difficult to consistently eat enough fruits and vegetables. Note: I said "boost." You want to work toward shifting your dietary choices to more fruits and vegetables. In the meantime, a formula such as this can help your body get what it needs along the way and can then augment once you arrive at your food goals.

If your multivitamin formula just doesn't make the grade or if you aren't taking one at all, it's time to go out and get one. Hop on down to your local supplement store or just call us at the Center at (888) 771-5166. We have this product available and the others mentioned at our online store at www.aplaceofhope.com.

Optional BGD Road Trip

I recognize that some of you reading this book will have real challenges to taking and absorbing nutritional supplements. You may have a physical condition that compromises your body's ability to utilize or even digest supplements. If that is the case, I urge you not to give up. There are strategies you can use to assist your body in regaining the ability to absorb nutrients.

You may need to take digestive enzymes to help your body break down your food and supplements. It may mean taking healthy digestive bacteria, such as acidophilus and bifidus. These are the healthy little bugs that live in your digestive tract that happily spend their days breaking down the food you eat so it can be absorbed into your intestinal tract. They're happy little bugs, but they can be disrupted by an overgrowth of yeast in your system, called *Candida albicans*, which happens through the use of antibiotics, some medications, and chronic stress that suppresses the immune system and allows the yeast to grow.

Candida occurs naturally in the body. Certain factors such as overuse of antibiotics can cause an overgrowth of candida, which can lead to total body disruption. Symptoms of candida overgrowth can affect all the systems in the body. Here are some examples:

- Digestive—bloating, gas, constipation, diarrhea
- Skin—rashes, acne, eczema, athlete's foot, toenail fungus
- Mental—fogginess, depression, forgetfulness, confusion
- Nervous—anxiety, panic attacks, mood swings
- Musculoskeletal—muscle pain and weakness, joint pain, general stiffness, fibromyalgia
- HEENT—headaches, dizziness, chronic sinusitis, itchy ears and decreased hearing, thrush
- GYN—PMS, vaginitis (yeast infections)
- Other—sugar or carbohydrate cravings, weight gain/retention

The best test for candida is a simple blood test for IgG antibodies in the blood. Stool can also be tested as well as saliva. One can also test by eliminating yeast from the diet and evaluating if symptoms improve.

Adherance to a rigorous candida elimination diet along with a strong anti-candida herb formula is the best way to decrease candida back to normal levels. This can last anywhere from one month to six months, depending on severity. It is best to see a specialist to help you through this protocol and for general support.

If you have a disrupted digestive system, you may want to consult with a naturopathic physician, someone medically trained in the use of nutritional supplements and alternative treatments. If you don't have a naturopathic physician available where you live, more and more traditionally trained medical doctors are realizing the benefits of natural approaches to symptom relief and healing. These professionals are out there; you may need to call around to find them, however.

If you're unsure whether or not your body is utilizing nutrients properly, or if it's been awhile since you've had a physical examination, I urge you to set aside your objections and make that call. Let your physician know of your desire to live a healthier lifestyle and gain his or her partnership in achieving your goals. It's pretty routine nowadays for your physician to run a complete blood count (CBC) during physical examinations. This can give valuable information on cholesterol and glucose levels for heart disease and diabetes risks. You might also consider having a urinary metabolic profile (UMP) run. This report will let your physician know how well you are utilizing nutrients, highlighting problem areas to be addressed.

Your body is an incredible machine, finely tuned by God to encase the spirit He gave you and His Spirit who indwells you. The fuel for this machine is equally complex and elegant in design. If some of you are having difficulty agreeing to take the time to understand nutrition and supplements, consider it an exercise in expanding your knowledge of God. The admonition in Romans 1:20 is for all of us: "For since the creation of the world God's invisible qualities—his eternal power and divine nature—have been clearly seen, being understood from what has been made, so that men are without excuse." Within the knowledge of your body and what it takes to feed it, fuel it, and function lie God's eternal power and divine nature. While it is perfectly appropriate to explore the stars and plumb the depths of the ocean for knowledge of God and confirmation of His power and nature, don't overlook the miracle that literally is around you, your body, which He designed. You'll learn about yourself, about God, and be blessed in your effort.

Father, thank You for the complexity You designed into my body. Help me to understand how to fuel it properly. Give me insight in the nutritional supplements I choose and how to use them. Never let them substitute for the good food You designed for my body to eat, but allow them to fill in the gaps to keep my body strong and healthy. Thank You for revealing Your truth to health-care professionals. Help me find those who are grounded in that truth. Amen.

Chapter 5

Fear-o-fat-o-phobia

> And at the end of ten days their countenances appeared fairer, and they were fatter in flesh, than all the youths that did eat of the king's dainties.
>
> —Daniel 1:15, ASV

> At the end of the ten days they looked healthier and better nourished than any of the young men who ate the royal food.
>
> —Daniel 1:15

The different translations of this Bible verse point perfectly to our fear-o-fat-o-phobia. Instead of translating the phrase "they were fatter in flesh," as the American Standard Version does, the New International Version reads they were "better nourished." The ASV was published in 1901. The NIV came out in 1973. In 1901, "fatter in flesh" still sounded pretty good. By 1973, "fatter in flesh" just wouldn't do anymore. It didn't convey the same positive connotation. Instead, the phrase was changed to "better nourished." Doesn't "better nourished" sound better to you? I think all of us would like to be "better nourished." Heaven forbid, however, that anyone should come up to me and say I looked "fatter in flesh."

This is the fat chapter. And we're actually going to use the word *fat*; we're not going to hide from it. After all, when people are overweight, the *weight* that they're *over* isn't muscle or bone; it's fat. Overweight is overfat. Those who are obese aren't obese because they're carrying around an extra leg or arm; they're obese because they are carrying around extra fat. We're obsessed with a word we don't want to use. I just think it's time we talked about it honestly. I think it is time we learn to put fat into perspective in our lives and lifestyles.

Your body as God designed it is not a body without fat. *Fat* isn't a bad word to God. Scripture uses it in a positive connotation in the Daniel verse, no matter how we try to interpret our way around it. (The King James Version uses the same phrase as the ASV, "fatter in flesh," while the New American Standard Version doesn't mince words and says simply, "they were fatter." End of story.) Back then, skeletal thinness was a cause for alarm, not acclaim, and it was associated with illness, not health.

God doesn't share our fat phobia. He created it in animal and plant forms. He even incorporated it into His system of sacrifices, requiring the people of Israel to offer up to Him both animal fat (He really liked the aroma of animal fat burning on the altar, saying it was very pleasing) and plant fat in the form of olive oil. The fat portion of the offering was special. In Genesis 4:4, in the first recorded offering to God, Abel brought the fat portions from some of his first flock, and the Lord looked at him with favor. God created the fat portions of our bodies. The body God designed for each of us is a body that includes a healthy balance of fat and that consumes fats as part of a healthy diet.

Yes, this is the fat chapter, and you're going to learn to appreciate fat. In order to help you get over this cultural hump, I'm going to talk about society's obsession with fat and how *fat* has become a bad word. I'm also going to talk about fat within the context of nutrition. You need to understand the forces at work around this concept of fat, both on your body and in your food, because obsession with fat has become both an idol and a trap.

If *fat* is always a negative word to you, it will be more difficult for you to grasp the next body God designed concept: **(D)—Discard fad diets**. The wisdom of the world says fad diets are good because diets will help you lose fat, which is bad. The worldly equation is:

Diet=good, because fat=bad

The culture around us is going to argue vociferously against discarding fad diets. But you must not listen. If you allow yourself to be lured by the siren song of fad diets, you will find yourself on a crash course with poor health.

The Wisdom of This Age

This whole fat obsession thing rises up out of three distinct but interrelated axioms of the world's wisdom. This world we live in (meaning our little or not-so-little corner of the world) says the following:

- Youth is king!
- Thin is in!
- You can have it all!

These are worldly "truths," and they are not designed to set you free. Instead, they are designed to keep you enslaved.

Youth is king

Let's start with this one because it may seem the least obviously tied to fat. Other cultures venerate age and the wisdom gained through age. Our American culture venerates youth. Biblical times were not like today's Western culture. In the Old Testament, Job put it very succinctly when he said, "With aged men is wisdom, and in length of days understanding" (Job 12:12, ASV). Back then, growing older was considered to have advantages. Age brought wisdom, which was good.

Our culture, however, values youth. We are, after all, a production-driven society. When are people perceived to be most productive? When they're young. Our culture values youthful appearance. What happens to most people as they age? They get fatter. They start jobs, sit a lot, have babies, start drinking, stop playing sports, come under more stress, have the keys to their own cars so they don't have to walk anymore, have keys to their own cars so they can go through any drive-through they want—all of which translates into more fat. If we all want to look younger, then we must all look thinner. Thin is young. Productive is young. Thin is productive. Slowing down and getting fatter is age.

We are obsessed with looking younger. Which of us wakes up in the morning, looks in the mirror, sees the effects of our age, and says, "Yeah! Now that's what I'm talking about!" Instead, we get up, look in the mirror, see the effects of our age, and spend the next twenty or thirty or forty minutes attempting to correct, retard, hide, or gloss over those effects.

One of the effects of age is increased weight. As we age, we tend to get larger. OK, let's just call it what it is—*fatter*. After all, we're not usually getting larger because of putting on muscle or growing another two inches; we get larger because we put on more body fat. And we come to hate ourselves for it. Thus, our increasing age becomes a curse, not a blessing. That's worldly thinking, and it dishonors God.

Thin is in

For all of our cultural hysteria over fat—being fat, fat grams, trans fats, saturated fats, fatty acids, fat portions, liquid fats, solid fats, partially hydrogenated fats—we're fatter than ever. I remember looking at the cover of *National Geographic* several years ago. From a distance, all I could see was a picture of what looked like rolling hills or folds of fabric. Upon closer inspection, it turned out to be the undulating contours of human fat, a discreet side view of an ample abdomen. What looked like hills or fabric from a distance was the rolls of fat around some brave woman's middle. It was very artistically done, but you and I both know that many people would look at this picture, and at this woman, in utter disgust and revulsion. Why? Because she dared show what so many of us try so hard to hide—fat.

We would never want anyone to come up to us and say, "You look great! Much fatter in flesh than last time I saw you!" That may have been a compliment in Daniel's day, but it is an insult in ours. Such a comment would send us straight to Curves or Baskin-Robbins—and sometimes, paradoxically, to both. (In my little town, the local Curves is actually next to the local Baskin-Robbins. Go figure.)

Since women are far less immune to the cultural biases that surround fat, let's just talk about what this fat phobia has meant for women. When you look at the curves of Marilyn Monroe in the 1940s or the healthy figure of Doris Day in the 1950s, you can see that the ideal of feminine beauty wasn't always in sync with a diagnosis of anorexia. These women were normal-sized women, admired for their hourglass shapes.

Then something happened in 1966. Womanly figures became passé, pushed out by a sixteen-year-old English phenomenon named Lesley Hornby. Her nickname was Twigs because of her skinny legs. What started as a childish snipe at knobby knees morphed into the name of the first true supermodel—Twiggy. With her enormous eyes, banana body, and androgynous look, Twiggy muscled the previous standards of beauty right off the catwalk. Naturally thin, fashions flowed off Twiggy without catching on any unnecessary bumps or lumps, so clothiers loved her. When she retired from modeling at the ripe old age of twenty, she said it was because she was tired of being a human clothes hanger. Twiggy got out of the game before the '60s ended. The rest of world, however, just kept right on going. Thin was in. Youth was in.

Now, more than forty years later, anorexic teenage models are dying of heart attacks and other complications of anorexia after living for months on lettuce leaves and Diet Coke. Fast-forward from 1966, and fashion models are being screened for BMI (body mass index) in order to prove they're not too thin for the runway. At a recent show in Madrid, 30 percent of those who showed up were turned away because of their emaciation.[1]

Models, of course, are not to blame; we are. That's right, the blame lies with you and me and this culture we live in and allow to mold our thoughts, attitudes, and actions. I'm certainly not going to blame Twiggy, but I figure somewhere about forty years ago we started down a path to collective loathing for body fat. It seems ironic, of course, that during the same time frame we began to revere the uberthin, we began to pack on the pounds as a society. It's a case of cultural masochism in which we revere those who epitomize a standard we're unwilling to emulate. It may also be a case of cultural envy in which we revere those who seem able to achieve what we're fearfully sure we cannot.

This is the world's definition of a paradox. It's also what God calls foolishness. We read in 1 Corinthians 3:19, "For the wisdom of this world is foolishness in God's sight." Our world places value and worth on youth and thinness for a body that ages and grows fatter. This is not a win-win situation for us.

You can have it all

Also around the 1960s, the concept of liberation came into play. Youth was to be liberated from antiquated morality. Free love, free sex, free drugs. Coming into adulthood meant writing your own rules, setting your own course, doing things your own way. Some of us set our course toward the all-you-can-eat buffet. The motto became, "If it feels good, do it." Well, for a whole lot of us now, eating prepackaged, processed convenience foods feels pretty good, so we do it. We actually *do* have it all. Our local grocery store, fast-food outlet, and convenience store are more than happy to provide it. We can have it all—all just isn't good for us.

It Doesn't Add Up

Do you see how skewed this equation has become? We're all supposed to strive to stay young or at least stay younger-looking. We're all supposed to strive to be thin. We're all supposed to be empowered to live our own lives and make our own decisions. But what if the way we choose to live our own lives and the decisions we make cause us to gain weight? What do we do then? The answer for far too many Americans is to continue to gain weight, year after year after year.

We put on weight and hate ourselves for it. We decide fat is not our friend; fat is our enemy. We think if we can eliminate all fat from our diets, we can be free from the fat around our bellies, butts, and thighs. We begin to look for "fat free" on all of our food choices, including salad dressing, chips, and cookies. As long as it says "fat free" on the chocolate cookies, we feel fine about watching television and eating the entire box.

There's just one problem with that line of thinking. The extra fat on our bodies is not necessarily related to the fat in our diet. Fat is stored excess energy. When we eat more calories than our bodies need to perform each day, the excess is stored as body fat. Now, it may be true that doughnuts are really hips in the larval stage, but that's more a function of the calories than the fat. If we eat 500 calories a day more than we need—even if that 500 calories is made up of fat-free products—we're still going to end up with an extra pound of body fat for the week. By depriving ourselves of healthy fats, our food becomes less appealing and less filling. We end up eating more and more in order to be satisfied. So, instead of helping us lose weight, our obsession with fat actually causes us to gain it.

Fat Facts

People need fat to live. Children need fat to be healthy and grow. Babies need fat to develop. Society's disgust with body fat has spread out (no pun intended) to encompass fat in general. That's more of the world's wisdom talking, which is foolishness. It's time to get the skinny on fats and learn which fats are good for you and which ones aren't. Then you can begin to make better choices about what you eat. Different fats react in the body in different ways. The body God designed for you doesn't require you to give up all fats forever. It does, however, require you to choose fats that will work *with* your body, not against it.

Essential fatty acids—what's the first word in that phrase? *Essential.* Yes, some fats are essential. Merriam-Webster's Online Dictionary has this definition of *essential*: "being a substance that is not synthesized by the body in a quantity sufficient for normal health and growth and that must be obtained from the diet." There are certain fats that are essential for normal health and growth. God designed you to need certain types of essential fats. These essential fatty acids are also known as omega fatty acids, the best-known being omega-3 and omega-6 fatty acids.

Omega-3 fatty acids

Let's talk about omega-3s first, of which there are three major types: alpha-linoleic acid (ALA), eicosapentaenoic acid (EPA), and docosahexaenoic acid (DHA). (Don't worry, there won't be a quiz at the end of this chapter, and you won't be expected to spell these, let alone pronounce them properly. It is a good idea, however, to learn their alphabetic shorthand.)

Do you remember the dietary guidelines I talked about earlier? It's no coincidence that omega-3s are found in such dietary sources as whole grains, fresh fruits, vegetables, fish, olive oil, and garlic. EPA and DHA come from cold-water fish, and this is generally the source for supplements. But you can eat the fish (salmon, albacore tuna, halibut, herring, sardines, and mackerel) just as well.

Of course, every silver lining comes with a cloud, and the cloud in freshwater fish is heavy metal contamination. For several years, the American Heart Association has recommended people eat at least two servings of fish per week. Along with that recommendation comes a warning that children and pregnant and nursing women should watch the type of fish they eat to avoid the risk of mercury poisoning. You can always supplement with a fish oil capsule as long as you make sure the manufacturer guarantees their products are free of heavy metal contamination.

Luckily, the body can take ALA and make EPA and DHA also. (God is the originator of backup systems—just think about your kidneys.) ALAs are found in flaxseed and flaxseed oil, soybeans and soybean oil, canola oil, as well as in pumpkin seeds and walnuts.

This kind of fat is really, really good for you. (If that makes you cringe, just read through the list below. It's very impressive and should help you to begin to understand that certain fats are good.) Essential fatty acids are not the current equivalent of snake oil. The following list of benefits of omega-3s came from an article put out by the University of Maryland Medical Center, Center for Integrative Medicine.[2] These nutrients are well researched and widely accepted. Essential fatty acids have been shown to:

- Make HDL, or "good," cholesterol levels higher and reduce LDL, or "bad," cholesterol levels and triglycerides.
- Lower blood pressure, especially for those who already have hypertension.
- Reduce the risk of heart disease and not just because of the first two reasons, although they are significant. There is research to show that omega-3s can help prevent plaque buildup in the arteries and the formation of blood clots. For those who have already suffered a heart attack, omega-3 supplements have been shown to help prevent death from subsequent heart attacks or strokes.
- Appear to reduce the risk of stroke as long as the amount taken is not more than 3 grams per day (a gram of essential fatty acids is roughly what you get from one serving of fish, which means you'd have to eat three servings of fish every day to put yourself outside of the healthy range). These substances help prevent arteries from clogging, and what's good for the heart is also good for the brain.

Additionally, studies have shown the following potential benefits from including essential fatty acids in your diet:

- If you're prone to diabetes, you may have high triglyceride and low HDL levels because they tend to go hand in hand. Since omega-3s help with these other two conditions, chances are they'll be good for you if you're diabetic. Be sure to use EPA and DHA sources, however, since some diabetics aren't able to convert ALA into a more readily used form. (Of course, you will want to discuss any dietary changes with your doctor first.)

- Omega-3s help people who are involved in a weight-reduction program that includes exercise and a low-fat diet. The fat these people do eat should be in the omega-3 category. This type of program helps maintain lower blood sugar and cholesterol levels.
- These fats have been shown to decrease inflammation. Because of this, there is research to suggest those with arthritis can benefit from omega-3s.
- EPA also helps with bone strength, assisting those with osteoporosis by boosting blood levels of calcium and helping to transport that calcium into bones.
- These fatty acids assist with cellular communication, as they are a component of cell membranes. When our cells can talk to each other better, we feel better; we feel happier and more upbeat. Eating a diet rich in omega-3s has been shown to decrease feelings of depression.
- Encouraging work is being done into identifying a link between omega-3s and reduced symptoms of bipolar disorder. According to this University of Maryland report, the UCLA School of Medicine is involved in a study to determine if such a correlation exists, as was shown in a similar but smaller study.

- It's possible that a link between a reduction in symptoms of ADHD and the use of omega-3 fatty acids may be determined.
- Because these essentially fatty acids help reduce inflammation, they have been used with burn victims to promote healing.
- When used in conjunction with medications, omega-3s may help those with inflammatory bowel disease (ulcerative colitis or Crohn's disease).
- For asthma sufferers, omega-3s may help reduce inflammation and increase lung capacity.
- EPA and DHA have been found to be correlated to a reduction in the risk for macular degeneration. In the same study, however, ALA appeared to increase the risk.
- A study in Denmark showed that a diet rich in omega-3s appeared to help reduce the symptoms of menstrual pain.
- Omega-3s appear to reduce the risk of colon cancer in the early stages. However, once the cancer has metastasized, omega-3s may promote the growth of cancer cells.
- Research is just beginning, but it looks promising that there may be a link between a diet rich in omega-3s and a reduction in the risk for breast cancer.
- EPA and DHA may retard the growth of prostate cancer, while ALA may promote it.

So, let's just take another look at our list of possible benefits for this essential fatty acid:

- Higher good cholesterol; lower bad cholesterol
- Lower blood pressure
- Reduced risk of heart disease
- Reduced risk of stroke
- Help for cholesterol levels in diabetics
- Assistance in weight-loss programs
- Reduced symptoms of arthritis
- Increased calcium to counter osteoporosis
- Help with depression
- Help with bipolar disorder
- Help for ADHD
- Benefits for those with eating disorders
- Promotion of healing for burns
- Help with inflammatory bowel disease (IBD)
- Help with asthma
- Reduced macular degeneration
- Reduced menstrual pain
- Reduced risk of colorectal cancer in the early stages
- Reduced risk of breast cancer
- Reduced risk of prostate cancer

This study also suggests that further research is needed, but say there's evidence to indicate that omega-3s could be beneficial in the treatment of certain types of infections, for ulcers, migraine headaches, early labor, emphysema, psoriasis, glaucoma, Lyme disease, lupus, and panic attacks. There was a warning, however, that increased consumption of omega-3s could increase bleeding. So individuals who have a tendency to bruise easily should consult with their physicians regarding use of omega-3 supplements.

Even with the warnings, I think you'll agree that omega-3s are good fats. These are fats you want to include in your diet. And since it may not be possible for you to get the amounts you need from the foods you eat, you may want to take EPA and DHA in supplement form. To aid you in determining which brand to buy, the University of Maryland Medical Center recommends 540 to 720 mg of EPA per day and 360 to 480 mg of DHA per day. This is equivalent to two or three servings of fish per week. Instead of taking supplements, you could also—gasp!—eat fish several times a week. Just don't make it tuna for every meal because of the mercury warnings.

Omega-6 fatty acids

OK, those were the omega-3s, not to be confused with the omega-6s. (The difference between omega-3s and omega-6s has to do with the molecular structure, which is so confusing it would take a biochemist to understand it. But if you're brave and did very, very well in high school or college chemistry, you're welcome to join in the fun on Wikipedia and read all about it. Go to http://en.wikipedia.org/wiki/Essential_fatty_acid.) To make it easier to remember, think fish and flax for omega-3s. For omega-6s, think meat and oils.

Omega-6s are found in meat and also in oils such as evening primrose oil, borage oil, and black currant seed oil.[3] Omega-6s come from linoleic acid (LA), which the body converts into gamma-linoleic acid (GLA), which is broken down even further into arachidonic acid (AA). The only reason I'm giving all these letters to you is so you'll know what they are when you go to the supplement store in search of a good fatty acid supplement (in this chapter's BGD Road Trip).

The list of positive and potential positives for omega-6s is similar to those for the omega-3 fatty acids. Here are some conditions specific to the benefits found from omega-6s:

- For those with diabetes, GLA and evening primrose oil may help with peripheral neuropathy, which is the lack of feeling and circulation that can come from diabetes.
- GLA may be helpful for those with dry-eye or dry-mouth syndromes.
- GLA and EPA may help maintain or increase bone mass, to help those suffering from osteroporosis.
- Evening primrose oil and GLA may be helpful for menopausal women who experience hot flashes.
- GLA may be helpful in alleviating premenstrual symptoms, such as breast tenderness, swelling and bloating from liquid retention, and feelings of depression and irritability.
- Omega-6s might help those who suffer from eczema or other skin conditions. The research is contradictory but may be worth looking into with your physician.
- Evening primrose oil may help reduce the severity of alcohol cravings and prevent damage to the liver.
- Omega-6s may reduce allergic reactions in some people.

The research regarding omega-6s does not appear to be as universally accepted or conclusive as research done about omega-3 fatty acids. However, new studies are adding to the scientific data on a regular basis. What does seem to be pretty well documented is the need to balance the intake ratio of omega-3s to omega-6s. Our typical diet in this country leans heavily toward omega-6s, probably due to our high consumption of meat. We tend to consume from eleven to thirty times more omega-6s than we do omega-3s. The more desirable ratio appears to be one to four times as many omega-6s as omega-3s.

The recommended dosage for adults hasn't been established yet. The University of Maryland article put it at 480 mg per day of GLA for those with diabetes, while those with rheumatoid arthritis were recommended to take 1,400 mg per day of GLA. It did say, however, that up to 2,800 mg per day appeared to be "well tolerated."

Omega-6s come with a greater list of precautions than omega-3s, especially in how they may interact with prescription medications. If you take ceftazidime, cyclosporine, anti-inflammatories such as ibuprofen, phenothiazines to treat schizophrenia, or are undergoing chemotherapy for cancer, you will want to check with your physician regarding the use of GLA and evening primrose oil.

There are several oils that contain essential fatty acids. Probably the most well known is olive oil; it's also my favorite for cooking. You can also find essential fatty acids in soybean oil, canola oil, and flaxseed oil. Oils are fats that stay liquid at room temperature, unlike that chemically altered modern marvel Crisco that we talked about earlier. But not all oils are equal. The MyPyramid.gov Web site notes that there are two types of oils that are so high in saturated fats that they should be treated like solid fats: coconut oil and palm kernel oil. I venture to guess that if I opened up the cabinets of nine out of ten readers of this book, I would find no bootleg bottles of coconut oil or palm kernel oil. Instead, what I would find would be processed, packaged foods that contain these types of oils. By reading food labels, you can find out what types of oils are used during the manufacturing process. Watch out for any product that uses coconut oil or palm kernel oil.

Watch out also for fats that become solid at room temperature such as butter, margarine, Crisco, and animal fat. (Think of bacon grease as it cools in that old Crisco container.) Bacon grease congeals naturally. Crisco, of course, has to be coaxed through hydrogenation into becoming a solid mass. These truly are bad fats. I've already talked about how you should steer clear of hydrogenated fats. Animal fats contain cholesterol and should be eaten sparingly.

Monounsaturated and polyunsaturated fats

Many food labels now differentiate between types of fats (monounsaturated, polyunsaturated, and saturated fats) without any explanation. Monounsaturated fats are those with a molecular design of one double-bonded carbon atom (thus the "mono-" part). Monounsaturated fats are found in nuts and avocados, as well as olives, peanut oil, flaxseed oil, corn oil, and canola oil. These are naturally occurring fats and should be a part of your overall diet, within the guidelines set up through your meal-tracking worksheet. Don't be afraid of the occasional avocado in your salad!

Polyunsaturated fats have more than one double-bonded carbon atom on the molecule. ("More than one" equals the "poly-" part of the word.) Polyunsaturated fats are good for your cellular health. Most essential fatty acids are polyunsaturated fats. When looking at food labels, you want to see the fats made up of monounsaturated and polyunsaturated fats, as opposed to the next category, saturated fats.

Saturated fats

These fats are called "saturated" because their molecular structure is naturally saturated with hydrogen atoms. Saturated fats include butter, coconut oil, and palm kernel oil—the bad fats. They are also found in meats and dairy products such as cheese and cream. Because they can raise your cholesterol, you want to eat these types of fats sparingly.

Trans fats

We've already talked at length about our friend Crisco. Trans fats are found in small quantities in meat and dairy items, but most of the trans fats eaten today are from hydrogenated or partially hydrogenated oils used in processed cookies, crackers, and baked goods. These are the really bad fats because their molecular structure makes them stick to your arteries like peanut butter sticks to the roof of your mouth. They are the modern-day culinary pariahs, as evidenced by the amount of denial used in packaging. Since there are so many good fats available to you, it is a good idea to eliminate trans fats from your diet as much as possible.

Cholesterol

Most of us probably know cholesterol by its Jekyll and Hyde personalities—HDL, the "good cholesterol," and LDL, the "bad cholesterol." But did you know that the membranes of your cells are made of cholesterol? Cholesterol is also important in the utilization of fat-soluble vitamins, such as vitamin D, and it's an important component in sex hormones. So, cholesterol is actually a good thing, but, like most good things, you can have too much of it. In our diets, cholesterol is obtained through eating eggs, beef, and poultry. A little bit is good, but you need to watch the amount you consume, especially if your body is genetically prone to manufacture lots of bad cholesterol and not so much good cholesterol.

One Sheet to the Wind

I've been talking about good fats, bad fats, and really bad fats, but no fat is really bad in and of itself. It's just that if you overdo the amount you consume, the amount becomes bad. In moderation (used "sparingly," as the food pyramid says), these are fine. No food is inherently more "righteous" than another. God created creamy milk and coconuts and palm kernels. You may need a vision similar to Peter's (see Acts 10); you need to see a sheet full of all kinds of fats. You need to hear God say that all of them are acceptable to eat. Your challenge is to know what you're eating, when you're eating, how to eat appropriately, and in what combination.

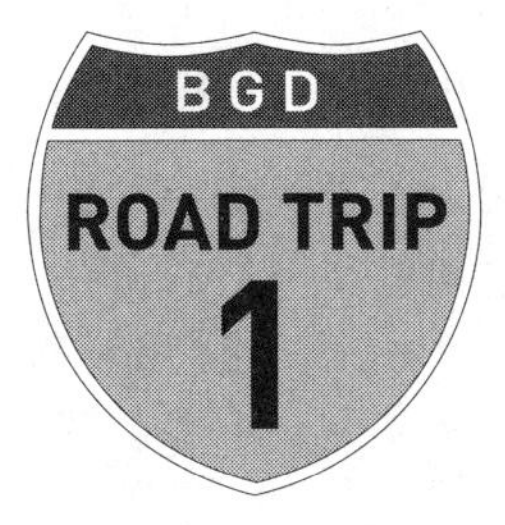

This time it's back to the kitchen and pantry cupboard. You've already taken a look at the packaging of the foods you eat. Hopefully by now you're starting to make some different choices, opting for more whole foods and less fragmented ones. Reality, though, suggests that you'll still have a certain amount of those brightly packaged, processed gems in your cupboard. Time to put another nail in the coffin. I want you to take out these packages, as well as any of the other foods with a label in your kitchen, and take note of the amounts of trans fats and monounsaturated, polyunsaturated, and saturated fats. What percentages are shown on these labels? How quickly can you get to 100 percent of your daily recommended servings? I imagine pretty quickly on some foods.

Use your meal-tracking worksheet to start keeping track of the fats you're consuming, especially the saturated kind. You're supposed to eat them "sparingly." Some of your favorite foods may simply be too "expensive" nutritionally to continue in the amounts of the past. This isn't to say you have to cut yourself off completely, but these foods must be shifted from a daily item on the list to an occasional one. Your divinely designed body needs a respite from a diet rich in saturated fats. It needs you to choose polyunsaturated oils, such as olive or canola oils.

Take a look at what's in your kitchen. How much saturated fat do these items represent? How many grams of trans fats are we talking about here? In your mind, think of a slab of lard or Crisco. Think of bacon grease coagulating into a solid white mass. That's what's happening in your arteries if you eat too much of these bad and really bad fats. Processed products high in these fats are not the friends of your arteries; they are the enemies.

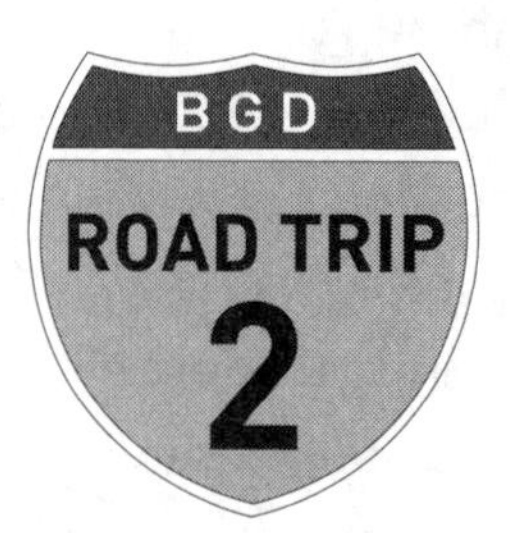

Are you now convinced that it's important to consume good fats, such as omega-3s (EPA and DHA)? Most people don't get the amount they need in their diets, so supplementation of these healthy fats is a good idea. Talk with your physician and find out if you're taking any prescription medication that could affect the amount of EPA and DHA you take. Ask about the ratio of EPA and DHA that is right for you. If your physician is skeptical, I recommend you see a naturopathic physician. The benefits of these supplements are becoming impossible to contradict, but some traditional medicine practitioners are not convinced.

Once you have the green light from your practitioner, head off to the supplement store and find a brand that has the right ratio of EPA and DHA for you. You don't have to buy the Cadillac of fish oil brands; retail outlets such as Costco carry good alternatives that come in large bottles to keep the unit price low. The two most important things you want to look for are the EPA/DHA ratios and to make sure the processing removes any heavy metals such as mercury. Oh, and while you're at Costco, pick up some salmon for dinner tonight and bottle of olive oil for your kitchen. It's perfectly fine to get these nutrients through natural food sources! ♡

Healthy Fats

I hope this chapter has helped you see that the body God created for you was designed to function best with good, healthy fats. Society's collective obsession with food labels that say "nonfat" and "fat-free" is not based on sound principles of nutrition. Body fat and fat in foods are part of God's creative design. Again, you must not let society's definitions and priorities propel you into unhealthy living and obsessive thinking. You must jettison your fear-o-fat-o-phobia. The more you know about your body and how it functions, the greater resistance you'll have to the kooky diet fads the media conjure up every couple of years.

Father, I give You praise for this body that You created. Help me to appreciate its beauty and unique nature as a gift from You. I confess I have not fed it properly in the past and have put more weight onto its frame than You intended. I commit to properly feeding this body You've given me. Thank You for providing such a variety of ways to eat healthy fats. Alert me to my patterns of eating that cause me to overindulge. I know from Daniel that rich foods do not lead to being better nourished. Give me strength to make the choices today that will nourish my body for a better tomorrow. Amen.

Chapter 6

The Pit of No Carbs in the Land of Right Now

> Then they said, "Come, let us build ourselves a city, with a tower that reaches to the heavens, so that we may make a name for ourselves and not be scattered over the face of the whole earth."
>
> —Genesis 11:4

Americans tend to be all-or-nothing, gotta-have-it-right-now kind of people. This includes our approach to dieting. Many of us decide "I have to lose this weight right now, or the world as I know it will end!" We believe the only way to achieve this goal is to undertake a frenzied course in tower-building, eating fifteen grapefruit a day, or never eating another carbohydrate again—ever.

This drive for immediate gratification is almost always coupled with sure calamity. Let's look at an example from the pages of the Bible. As you can read in this chapter's opening Scripture verse, the construction of the Tower of Babel began because people wanted to make a name for themselves and be bonded together by a common goal. These ambitions, in and of themselves, are not necessarily evil.

The problem is wanting to *do it myself*, which is the outcry of every two-year-old.

When it comes to eating, you probably want to *do it yourself*! You want to determine what, when, and how much you eat. After all, you're an adult, aren't you? Age is supposed to bring freedom to choose, isn't it?

Of course, God says that age is supposed to bring wisdom. For it is within the context of wisdom that freedom is fulfilled. Do you have the freedom in this country to eat whatever you want, in whatever quantity, whenever you want? The answer is yes, if you have the means to do so. (And most of us do pretty well, judging by our waistlines.) Simply put, you have the freedom in this country to gain weight.

The more weight you gain, the more desperate you are to take the weight off. You want a solution to your dilemma, but, once again, you want to choose the solution that works best for you, that feels most comfortable, and that has the least amount of lifestyle change—a pill, an appetite suppressant, a metabolic energizer. You want something quick, simple, relatively painless, and extraordinarily effective. You want a short-term fix to a long-term issue. You're willing to deprive yourself for a short amount of time—until summer's over, until the high school reunion has passed, until the holidays, until your daughter's married and off on her honeymoon. You tell yourself that what you need is the right diet and the pounds will melt off, the unsightly fat will be gone, and you will have freedom!

Crazy About Diets

Americans are really crazy about diets. Just look at the magazine rack at your local grocery store. What's on the front of almost every cover? An attractive, thin, ubiquitous (yes, that word again) model with a story about how you too can lose thirty pounds in eight weeks.

Eight weeks is probably the average desperation phase. You realize about eight weeks before your high school reunion that you haven't lost the twenty pounds you swore you would when the invitation first arrived. You realize about eight weeks before your daughter's wedding (or your own) that the stress of the preparations has caused you to put *on* five pounds. You realize in the spring that summer's right around the corner and you're nowhere near ready to be seen in shorts, let alone a bathing suit. Now you've entered the desperation phase, where you're willing to try anything, suspend any level of belief, and attempt the latest diet gimmick, no matter how incredible the claims may be.

Allow me to be unequivocal—diets don't work. They may produce some results in the short term, but they have no staying power in the long term. What *does* work is changing your habits and lifestyle choices slowly over time (back to baby steps). The only way to do that is to face up to your fears, including fear-o-fat-o-phobia and the mentality of "I have to lose weight right now or the world as I know it will end!" and start making healthy choices about food.

Changing unhealthy eating patterns is a little like making the *Titanic* change its course. Course changing needs to be done slowly over time with great consistency and concentration. It also, by definition, means you're heading out in a new direction. If you turn the *Titanic*, you have to want to change course. Most of us, however, don't want to change course. What we'd really like is a short diversion. These short diversions are called diets, and they come in a couple of different forms.

The "if a little is good, a lot is better" approach to dieting

This one is like the grapefruit diet I alluded to earlier. Someone, somewhere, decided that grapefruit was good for dieting. (This discovery was attributed to the Mayo Clinic, but I doubt that's where it actually originated. In fact, if you go to the Mayo Clinic's homepage and type in "grapefruit" in the search box, you get a rather interesting article detailing how grapefruit, as well as tangelos and Seville oranges, actually interfere with a variety of prescription medications from Zoloft to Viagra.) However this one started, the theory is that if one grapefruit a day is good for dieting, then many grapefruits a day should be *great* for dieting.

I seem to remember that awhile back there was also an avocado diet. It didn't last long, probably because avocados, while they are delicious and good for you in small quantities, are pretty calorie rich. Unlike the avocado diet, the grapefruit diet still has some adherents. It promised a large amount of weight loss in a short amount of time. A phenomenon of the '80s, it seems to be cycling back through as these things tend to do every twenty-five years or so.

The "if a little is good, a lot is better" diet fails to incorporate a key concept in healthy eating: moderation. The body God designed for you was made to respond best to foods eaten in moderation. Even good foods need to be eaten in moderation, or you will end up dealing with the next dieting diversion.

The "safe foods" approach to dieting

In my work with those overcoming eating disorders as well as people of normal weight, I find this "if a little is good, a lot is better" sentiment to be very common. When this mind-set is taken to extremes, it turns into the "safe foods" approach to dieting. Foods like grapefruit become a "food cocoon" in which the person feels safe from negative consequences. People choose safe foods because they believe the food is going to help them lose weight because it won't cause them to gain weight.

Safe foods are not chosen on a rational basis. One of the anorexic models who died in 2007 decided that lettuce was a safe food. Why did she consider it safe? Because eating lettuce leaves exclusively will cause a person to lose weight. She considered losing weight to be safe for her career goals; gaining weight was unsafe. Was eating lettuce leaves really "safe" for her? No. In losing weight, she lost her life.

Safe foods neglect to take into account another key concept in healthy eating: variety. God designed your body to function best when fed a wide variety of foods. He has shown His creativity and love for you in the cornucopia of foods He has provided: fruits, vegetables, grains, fish, poultry, meats, and dairy products. However, instead of looking to the Designer for direction, you may be tempted to stick to foods you consider safe. You think of them as manna from heaven—something you can eat every day. But unlike the miraculous manna provided for the Israelites in the wilderness, these foods provide an illusion of safety, but all the while they are imprisoning you.

Although you probably don't think about it, when you choose safe foods, you are actually operating from the same motives as the people who were building the Tower of Babel. You want to feel safe, and you want to make a name for yourself. And the name you want to make is the name "righteous." If you eat grapefruit, you're safe; if you eat grapefruit, you're righteous. Even when you're shown that eating too many grapefruit isn't good for you and might even be harmful, you're not willing to give up being safe or righteous. These things become more important than truth.

I want to go back again to Peter's vision in Acts 10. The vision about unclean foods was a metaphor to show Peter that there are no impure or unclean people. However, I think it's instructive when considering the "safe foods" approach to dieting.

God knew that Peter would understand this metaphor because of the way Peter felt about "clean" or safe foods. The truth Peter needed to accept was that God was the final arbiter of clean and unclean. In Acts 10:15, the voice from heaven warned him, "Do not call anything impure that God has made clean." That includes both food and people.

Jesus said something similar. "'Are you so dull?' he asked. 'Don't you see that nothing that enters a man from the outside can make him "unclean"? For it doesn't go into his heart but into his stomach, and then out of his body.' (In saying this, Jesus declared all foods 'clean.')" (Mark 7:18–19). There you have it, the definitive statement: all foods are clean. There aren't some foods that are "righteous" and some that are "unrighteous" or unclean. God doesn't declare some foods safe and some unsafe; we do that. God says He's given us a bounty of foods to eat and enjoy in moderation.

So, if you see a diet that touts the "miracle" of eating an abundance of one kind of food all the time, steer clear. If you want to eat a grapefruit now and again, go ahead (after checking first with your physician and the Mayo Clinic).

The "better life through pharmaceuticals" approach to dieting

This is one of my all-time favorite diet diversions. If you've ever suffered insomnia or had the misfortune to have nothing to do but watch cable television on a Saturday afternoon, you know what I mean. These are the diets that come in pill form, and their ads make liberal use of the words *miracle* and *amazing results*. One gelatin capsule or time-release tablet, one dietary supplement or appetite suppressant claims to "melt fat" or enable you to "eat whatever you want and still lose weight." Deep down, don't you want to be able to take a pill or ingest a miracle supplement and still lose weight while enjoying your chocolate cake for breakfast? I know I do!

The "better life through pharmaceuticals" approach to dieting neglects another key component in healthy eating: consistency. A healthy weight is a product of a consistent lifestyle, one in which you regularly choose not to consume more fuel than you burn in activity.

More importantly, these types of diets can be dangerous. Many of these products artificially pump up your metabolic rate. At one time, many appetite suppressants contained an ingredient you may recognize by its street name: speed. That's right, these appetite suppressants were juiced up with amphetamines. When you artificially or pharmaceutically rev up your metabolism, it affects your heart and blood pressure. It's as shocking to your system as going from couch potato to running in the Boston Marathon all in one day. The positive benefit of being consistent with a healthy lifestyle is that it prepares your body gradually over time. Your metabolism is built up naturally instead of being shocked into overdrive by amphetamines.

The "self-flagellation" approach to dieting

Some of you may be unfamiliar with the term *self-flagellation*. This was the thirteenth- and fourteenth-century practice of beating yourself with whips as penance for sin. It was a form of beating (literally) God to the punch. In other words, if I hurt myself for the bad I've done, maybe God will consider it enough and not punish me further. This practice was eventually outlawed by the Catholic Church and, seen through the lens of history, appears to us now to be both barbaric and utterly useless for atonement of any kind. That doesn't mean we don't still do it, however.

Self-flagellation diets surface on Monday right after a weekend of caloric excess. It's the "I'll start my diet on Monday" philosophy—or for those who prefer a scriptural reference, it's the "Let us eat and drink for tomorrow we die" philosophy (found in Isaiah 22:13 and 1 Corinthians 15:32). If you're like most people, you concentrate on the eating and drinking part, and then you attempt to put off the dying—or dieting—part.

Self-flagellation diets are those that have you eating less than half of the calories needed each day to maintain your weight. They're meant to get immediate, obvious results. They are, in essence, self-imposed starvation or near starvation. Your body doesn't respond well to threats of this kind. Go on a starvation diet, and your body will beat *you* to the punch because it will go into starvation mode. In starvation mode, your body turns down its internal thermostat and *reduces* your metabolic rate. Sure, you're taking in less calories, but your body responds by needing less. Your metabolism drops; your energy level drops; your body temperature drops; your fatigue level increases.

You can go back and forth with your body like this for a while and can actually lose weight. Here's the problem, however. At some point, inevitably, you'll go back to eating more calories. But your body is still at the depressed metabolic level. So, even if you don't eat as many calories as before, your metabolic demand has dropped, so you'll actually gain back the weight plus more. This may be why you feel your body is out to get you. Your body metabolism seems to have become the enemy.

To be fair, it wasn't your body that declared war on you. Rather, it is just acting in accordance to God's design. Your body doesn't know this self-induced starvation level was entered into with your full and total cooperation. Therefore, it reacts to this as a crisis and marshals its preservation mechanism to protect your life and, as an unfortunate consequence, to protect your fat.

The only way to work *with* your body and not against it is to lose weight slowly over time. This is the next key component in healthy living: permanence. Don't believe that undertaking to live a healthy lifestyle is only for times of desperation or to make up for the "sins" of the all-you-can-eat buffet. Don't relegate it to a temporary status. If you live a healthy lifestyle only temporarily, you've deluded yourself, and you have negated any benefits you would have gained.

The "suspension of reality" approach to dieting

If you're like most people, you probably can't afford to hire a personal chef to prepare all of your meals to make sure you're eating the foods you should in the appropriate quantities. The rich and famous can, but most of us aren't rich and famous. No live-in chefs for you or me. However, there are several popular diets available today that offer a shadow of this. For a fee, you can sign up for these diet plans, which aren't expensive in and of themselves. The real money is made through the purchase of the requisite meals. You can have breakfast, lunch, dinner, and snacks mailed to your home. How exciting it must be to receive an entire week's worth of food in a large cardboard box.

I call these diet plans the "suspension of reality" approach because having other people prepare your food every day isn't something that can be sustained. Eventually, you have to return to terra firma and deal with the reality of your kitchen, your cupboard, and your refrigerator. At some point, you'll need to venture forth to your local grocery store for more than batteries and laundry soap.

It's not that I find no value whatsoever in this type of diet. I think they give some people a "reprieve" from their battle with what and how much to eat. They provide an artificial structure so people can concentrate on other aspects of their overeating. During this artificial respite, hopefully the person is coming to grips with his or her dependency patterns surrounding food.

Unfortunately, I think the more common scenario is to cooperatively eat the food that has been sent but with occasional self-justified snacks thrown in. I mean, after all, if you're losing weight eating these prepackaged meals, which are really pretty skimpy compared to what you were eating before, there ought to be enough "wiggle room" in there for a bowl of ice cream, a candy bar, or a big, thick chocolate shake with whipped cream and a cherry on top, right?

This highlights a key concept for a healthy lifestyle—sustainability. It is not good for your body to undergo the ebb and flow of yo-yo diets. Up twenty, down twelve, up twenty-seven, down thirty, up ten, up seven, down five, up twelve. Slow and steady wins the race; sustainability sets the pace.

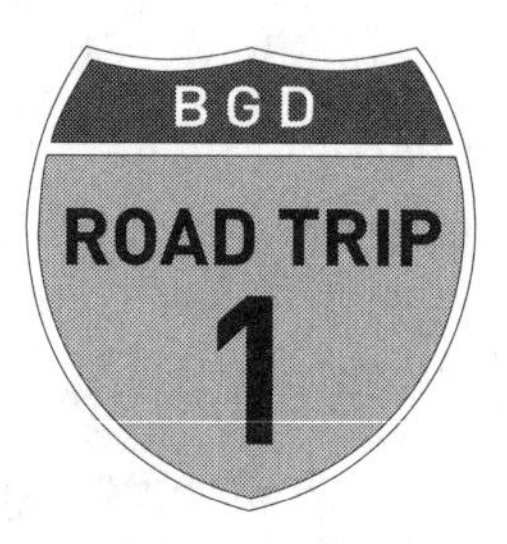

For this road trip, you're going to take mental journey back into your past. I venture to guess this isn't the first diet book you've picked up. You've probably tried one, two, three, or more of the approaches I've discussed to get the weight off! Am I right?

In this chapter, I've explored a variety of diet diversions that have been tried and touted over the years. For your review, they are:

- "If a little is good, a lot is better" (think grapefruit diet)
- "Safe foods" (think lettuce leaves)
- "Better life through pharmaceuticals" (think amphetamines)
- "Self-flagellation" (think Monday morning)
- "Suspension of reality" (think premade meals)

Through looking at the fallacies in these diet methods, we've talked about some key concepts of what it takes to really effect long-term weight loss and health. Those were:

- Moderation (fast and furious works for cars, not for weight loss)
- Variety (one food does not fit all day)
- Consistency (slow and steady wins the race to weight loss)
- Permanence (all-or-nothing diets leave you with nothing)
- Sustainability (losing weight is up to you, not up to a freezer box)

I'd like you to think back through the years at all the ways you've used to gain weight. That's right, I said *gain weight*, not *lose weight*. Most of us have pretty specific ways we've developed that lead to increased weight. It may be indulging in that "guilty pleasure" on a regular basis. It may be trading your roller skates for a TV remote. It may be "eating like there's no tomorrow" for the past twenty years. Start at the point you realized you were carrying around more weight than was normal for others your age. Was that in grade school? High school? College? What changed? What habits did you pick up that contributed to the weight gain?

OK, now think back to when you first started expending some effort at losing weight. How old were you? What sorts of things did you do back then to lose weight? Ask yourself, are those ways still effective today? (I'll talk more about that in chapter

10, the aging chapter, but I want you to start asking the question now.)

Take a look at the ways you've used to lose weight in the past. Since no one but you is going to see this, go ahead and name names. If you've used name-brand diets before, write them down. Now rate them for their effectiveness. Did they work in the short term? Did they work in the long term? Did you lose weight? Did you feel better? Were they a healthier way to eat? Some of these may have had some positives. Go ahead and feel free to put those down as well as the negatives.

Which one of the diet diversions I outlined did each of these fall into? If one doesn't really match up, can you come up with a name for it yourself? What are its flaws? Why didn't it work? What key concept or concepts were missing?

No, this is not meant to be mental self-flagellation. Rather, we're on a mission of discovery. By finding out what doesn't work, we come closer to finding out what does.

Finding Your Keys

I don't know about you, but I'm always losing my keys. I have keys to my house, to our cars, and to various doors and drawers and cabinets at my office. You'd think that with as many and how clunky they are, I could easily tell where I put them down. The sad fact is that I can't; I lose them all the time. It's being on autopilot that's to blame. I set them down in a mindless state while concentrating on something else, and when it comes time to use them, I can't for the life of me figure out where I put them. It would help, of course, if I put them in the same place consistently. Then, whenever I needed them, I'd know right where to go to find them.

Many people have the same challenge with the key concepts of healthy living. You have them in your toolbox; you know what they are. You've probably been carrying them around for a while. You just can't seem to find them when you need them.

For the rest of this chapter, you're going to design a "place" for all of these key concepts. You're going to discover what a healthy diet looks like for you.

You've already started down that path by tracking what you eat each day. You're becoming more aware of the actual content of the foods you eat and working toward incorporating more and more whole foods into your choices. You're also becoming more aware of your food patterns. I want you to reinforce the good patterns and begin to incorporate more of them.

Now it's time to get really serious about following your meal-tracking worksheet. This is your road map toward a healthier lifestyle. Using your meal-tracking worksheet will help you avoid the danger of diet diversions.

By following the guidelines listed, you'll automatically be partaking moderately of the foods most of us eat too much of—sweet and fatty foods. These are in the "oils and discretionary calories" category. While you can still have some of these foods, the caloric total is fairly low, so you'll need to cut down on the portion size. It doesn't mean you can't have your favorite cookie. You can, so enjoy your one cookie, not six as before. Realistically, how much did you really pay attention to those six cookies? Didn't you eat them in a rush while driving or watching television or reading? This time, take time over that cookie and really enjoy it in the context of all the other foods you've eaten today.

There's one thing this plan is very good for, and that's variety, which is the second key concept I shared with you. It even goes so far as to give you goal totals for the week of the various types of vegetables. It's important to vary your vegetables because different types have different nutrients. Vegetables are powerhouses of nutrition, so you don't want to max out on carrots all the time and miss the benefits of broccoli or squash. If you're someone who has difficulty eating different types of vegetables, start small. These guidelines are goals for you to work toward, not a rigid rulebook you must adhere to perfectly right now (which would take you back to your all-or-nothing thinking). Give yourself permission to grow and adjust over time. Gradual progress is the key. You can find a realistic pace for yourself. (Standing still or going backward is not progress, however, so throw out that thought for what it is—an excuse.)

By using this plan, you'll be developing consistency. After awhile, food choices will become easier. You won't have to do so much calculation to figure out how much of which thing is going to work for you. Eating this way—with whole grains, fruits, vegetables, lean meats, fish, and lean dairy products—will become your norm. Consistency builds habits. Habits allow you to relax and develop a flow that will become second nature to you.

Right now, you have your meal-tracking worksheet up where you can see it and use it every day. At some point, you'll decide you don't really need to do that anymore. Be aware that when you reach this point, you'll probably begin to drift back into some old habits. That's when it will be time to pull it out again or print up a new one to remind yourself. Healthy eating isn't a diet. It isn't something you suffer through so you can fit into that dress or suit jacket for the reunion. Instead, you must accept healthy eating as your goal (and benefit) for the rest of your life.

You cannot leave it up to other people to prepare healthy food for you. You're going to need to take ownership of your life and your health, and you have to become an active participant in deciding what you will put into your mouth. If you live by yourself, you'll need to take your plan with you to the grocery store so you can be sure to have available the variety and types of food you need to eat. If you live with others, you'll need to encourage them to join in with you. But be prepared to take control of your own food if they refuse to choose a healthy lifestyle with you. Ultimately, what you eat and how much you eat are up to you. As an adult, no one is forcing too much food down your throat.

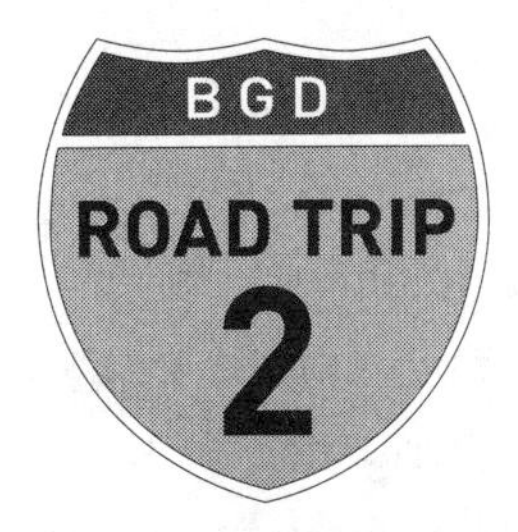

I can't say enough about the MyPyramid.gov Web site. This is an easy-to-understand, well-thought-out way to eat healthier and make positive changes. It is provided through the U.S. Department of Agriculture and is a product of the Center for Nutrition Policy and Promotion, which was established by the federal government in 1994. If you don't have access to a personal or public computer, I encourage you to call 1-888-7-PYRAMID (1-888-779-7624). Many government materials are available through the mail.

If you do have access to a computer, again, I encourage you to take the time to navigate around this site. If you haven't done so already, I encourage you to register at the Web site for MyPyramid Tracker. This is an online assessment of what you're eating and what physical activities you're engaged in that provides feedback about your progress and provides nutritional information.

Remember my discussion about establishing patterns over time? The MyPyramid Tracker allows you to input your food and your activity daily and follow the patterns for up to a year. This information is kept confidential. You establish a user name and a password, and you'll have access to your information from any computer, whether you're home, away on business, or on vacation.

It's fine also if you choose not to go this route. But I do want you to work toward meeting your daily and weekly goals in feeding your body a healthy balance of foods. You will not be able to regain or maintain the body God designed for you merely by wishful thinking. You will have to make intentional choices. Your divinely designed body is not going to happen by means of a magic pill or the latest fad diet. Instead, it is going to come about by working through the physical realities God has designed into His creation.

I understand—believe me, I understand—that many of our food choices and food habits have very little to do with nutrition and a great deal to do with emotional, spiritual, and physical factors. Next we're going to get into those areas and take a look at how they can adversely affect our ability to follow the simple keys of healthy eating and living.

For right now, I want you to agree with me that eating this way is what you need to do today—not Monday, not next week, but today. You've had your printout up on your fridge or cabinet for a while now, and you've been working toward putting them into practice. And for any of you who haven't started to put them into practice, step by baby step, the time really is now.

This is a diet that really does work—because it's not a diet; it's eating that honors the Creator of this body of yours. When you eat the way you want to, when you choose the latest miracle "fat-melting" diet, you say to God the very same thing the builders of the Tower of Babel said: "I want to do it myself." You cut God out of the picture of your body and your health.

Ultimately, the effort to build the Tower of Babel brought confusion to the earth. In the English language, "babble" is taken from the name *Babel*, and as I look over the myriad of diets marketed continually, I can't help but think that *babel* is really the right word for all of it. The clamor of all the claims, promises, pitches, and angles used to entice people to turn over their money in exchange for weight loss sounds like a cacophony if I ever heard one.

It's easy for your keys to get lost in the midst of all that confusion. Keep it simple, and focus on the key concepts:

- Moderation
- Variety
- Consistency
- Permanence
- Sustainability

These keys come from God's design. When you use these keys, they work with your body, not against it, and they allow you to live your life as God designed it to be lived, neither too fat nor too thin, but just right for the way He made you.

I can imagine you might be thinking, "First the fat chapter, now the diet chapter." If you're honest, you'll admit you really don't want to have to eat healthy to be healthy. You're sure that living this type of lifestyle means *deprivation*. Instead, you want to be able to eat the way you want and then have some diet or pill or potion make it all magically go away. It frightens you to think of living life without your comfort foods and predictable pleasures and eagerly anticipated rewards. I promise we will get into those areas later. For right now, I want you to accept your ambivalence toward the guidelines on your meal-tracking worksheet. I want you to accept the rebellion you feel when contemplating that it has to be this way forever. I want you to accept and commit to doing it anyway. If you never start, you'll never experience the benefits, including how good you can feel when you feed your body the way God intended you to feed it.

Trust God. Recognize your feelings of rebellion are nothing new to God. He's experienced them before. Do you remember what happened after the people of Israel were led out of captivity in Egypt by Moses? It didn't take the people long to start complaining and criticizing. As amazing as it sounds, they actually began to consider their old life in captivity and slavery to be better than their new life of freedom.

It is normal for human beings to resent change and fear the unknown. It is normal to rebel against doing the right thing. It's your sinful or fleshly nature coming to the forefront.

In the wilderness, God demonstrated His love for the people of Israel over and over again and personally led them into the Promised Land. There's a similar concept at work in your fear of striking out on a new culinary course. You know what to expect of your Twinkies and fried pork rinds and Crisco-fried chicken. You're familiar with your lattes and your ice cream and your french fries. Even though these foods have imprisoned you in excess weight, you still cry out for them when you're asked to change course.

Once again, God asks you to trust Him. When you feed your body the way it was created to be nourished, there are blessings to be realized. You can't experience them if you never risk changing your habits. Trust God and risk change.

Father, help me! Change is so hard! I confess I've made my own choices about food and allowed habits to build up, even when I knew they weren't healthy or good for me. I'm going to need Your help to change. I'm afraid of how hard it's going to be. I know Satan wants me to be enslaved to food, to continue to make the latest diet my idol instead of You. I want to be healthy and live a healthy life for You. Protect me from the schemes of Satan, and reveal to me daily the blessings of eating Your way. Keep me strong and making progress. Today, I give my food to You. Amen.

Chapter 7

The Proper Use of the Knife

And put a knife to your throat if you are given to gluttony.
Do not crave his delicacies, for that food is deceptive.
—Proverbs 23:2–3

When you've written on dieting, your life can become a bit complicated. For one thing, everyone expects you to be thin. After all, you're supposed to be an "expert," so certainly you must be thin yourself. The effectiveness of your writing is measured by the size of your own waist. Second, people sometimes react to a writer/counselor as they would to their parish priest or their neighborhood bartender. I call it the confession factor.

It's amazing how many people I meet who, after they find out what I do, feel compelled to make highly personal confessions. It wouldn't be so strange if it happened only in the private confines of my office. Instead, it can happen at social functions, sporting events, school programs—even at church. Sometimes I'm just trying to snag a cup of coffee before the service with my boys, and along comes someone who discloses a highly personal revelation—not only to me but also to any member of our church family within earshot. The need to "come clean" and to confess to another person is a very powerful force!

Because I work with eating disorders and disordered eating, one of the most common confessions I hear is gluttony. Now, people don't usually put it that way. I can't remember anyone actually coming up to me and saying, "I confess; I'm a glutton." However, people do tell me that they really eat too much or that they just can't seem to lose their excess weight.

Gluttony (excessive eating) is an antiquated word, and it's a biblical one. Ironically, in Christian social circles, drinking too much is considered a sin, while eating too much is just fine and dandy, especially at potlucks. I have found, however, that the bondage to food is as strong as, or stronger than, the bondage to drink. So, it always makes me feel a little queasy to see very large brothers and sisters carrying triple-portioned plates around in the church building. It's as inappropriate to me as having a happy hour after service.

So forget about what latest church fellowship activity seems to say about eating to excess, because the Scriptures are less charitable. In the Bible, gluttony is linked with drunkenness, disgrace, and laziness (Proverbs 23:21; 28:7; Titus 1:12). It's also one of the seven deadly sins as defined by Pope Gregory the Great in the sixth century. (The other six are pride, greed, lust, envy, anger, and slothfulness.)

At the root of gluttony is a lack of discipline. In fact, I would venture to say that although most people associate gluttony with being overweight, it's actually possible to be thin (remember those banana-shaped people from chapter 1?) and still be a glutton if you don't practice discipline in your eating habits.

So why is it such a struggle to be disciplined with our eating? It's not as if you haven't heard what's bad for you. You hear about it nearly every day from newspaper reports, breaking news on TV, and magazine articles. The government even has radio spots that extol the virtues of eating fruits and vegetables each day. We know what we need to do, and yet we don't do it. Many of us don't do it. A quick look at recent statistics reveals that gluttony is winning the day:

- One hundred twenty-seven million Americans are overweight with nine million morbidly obese.[1]
- For those over twenty-five years of age, 80 percent are overweight.[2]
- Almost 80 percent of all Americans fail to meet the recommendations for a basic activity level.[3]
- A fourth of us are completely sedentary.[4]
- Since 1990, there has been a 76 percent increase in the onset of type 2 diabetes in adults aged thirty to forty.[5]

The results are in, and it's not looking good for us as a country. Do you know they're even talking about a new word—*globesity*? Globe (world) + obesity = the worldwide problem of globesity. Take heart; it's not just us. Apparently there are significant parts of the world where obesity is a problem also. (Juxtapose this against the widespread starvation and malnutrition in other parts of the world.) Gluttony, while a problem in affluent American culture, is also a worldwide problem.

As I've said, it's not like we don't know what to do about it. We know that healthy eating requires us to avoid overeating and strive for proper nutrition. So why is it so hard to continue making good choices every day? Part of the reason is *we don't want to.* The other part is *it's hard to.* How can we learn to tame our urge to overeat without putting a knife to our throats?

Putting a knife to your throat seems a little harsh, doesn't it? I think Solomon was using a harsh statement to emphasize a harsh reality.

The harsh reality is the bondage that comes from gluttony or over-eating. The verse from Proverbs at the beginning of this chapter says it's possible to be "given to gluttony." With the high rates of obesity in this country and now the world, it appears that many of us are given to gluttony—and absolutely miserable about it. Miserable enough to want to confess to a veritable stranger in the church lobby. Miserable enough to pick up (one more!) diet book on the chance this one will work. God didn't make food to make you miserable. Instead, He meant it to bless you, but when you put food (or any gift from God) outside of His plan, you run into trouble.

Building Blocks to Health

Let me just say that I applaud you for getting this far in the book and in your resolve to live a healthier life. You're over halfway through the book, and I know you've had challenges to overcome. In this chapter and the next one, I am going to talk about some common hurdles and how to get around them.

I'd be willing to bet that in our journey together thus far, I've probably touched on at least one thing that mirrors what's happening in your life. You're aware of what to do but are having trouble pulling it off. That's OK. Let's take a minute and review the fundamentals to achieving the body God designed for you:

- **(A)—Accept yourself**
- **(B)—Be physically active**
- **(C)—Choose food wisely**
- **(D)—Discard fad diets**

Now we're going to talk about:

- **(E)—Eat for health**

You may ask, "Isn't eating for health a lot like choosing food wisely? Don't both of them deal with food?" Yes, but **(C)—Choose food wisely** is about understanding the types of foods you eat and making intentional choices. To **(E)—Eat for health**, you need to acknowledge a different side to the food equation—the fact that food wears a variety of hats in this culture and in your individual life. You should eat in order to fuel your body, but you eat for many more reasons than that. The next chapter is going to deal exclusively with *emotional eating*, which is huge in our culture. Right now, I'm going to talk about two other types of hurdles—one I call *ignorant eating* and the other I call *mindless eating.*

Isn't it good to know that you're ignorant and mindless? Now, before you take offense, just think about what good news that can be. If you're ignorant of something, all it means is that you need to learn something. Once you learn, you change from being ignorant to being *informed.* If you're doing something mindlessly, all it means is that you need to be clued in to the reality around you. Once you get clued in, you're not mindless anymore; you're *intentional.* Ignorant and mindless can be transformed into informed and intentional! Knowledge is a powerful thing. Allow it to affect you in a positive way so you can **(E)—Eat for health**.

Pounding out the portions

Ignorant eating has to do with portioning and serving sizes. This is one area where people always react with amazement when they actually become aware of what a real portion size is. Up to that *aha* moment, they've been living and eating in ignorance. When confronted with the truth, they'll ask in indignation: "Since when is one cookie a serving? Since when is three ounces of chicken a serving? Since when is eleven crackers a serving? Do you know how small that is? Who in their right mind eats only one cookie or eleven measly little crackers? And three ounces of chicken is, what, two bites? That's totally unrealistic!"

These are good questions because they get to the heart of society's ignorance about portions. When did this ignorance start? The answer, I think, is about fifty years ago.

I'm a baby boomer. For those of you who have never quite figured out where that term comes from, the *baby boom* refers to the sudden increase of children born right after World War II. Therefore, baby boomers are the generation of people who were born during the baby boom, which spans from 1945 to about 1960. I was born at the end of the boom, in 1959.

A few years before I was born, in 1955 to be exact, Ray Kroc opened the first McDonald's restaurant in Des Plaines, Illinois. It literally exploded onto the cultural landscape, bringing automation, uniformity, and french fries to millions. (Big Macs didn't show up until the 1970s. I can still sing the commercial from memory.) While McDonald's established the fast-food phenomenon and set the pace for years as an organization responsive to the demands of consumers, it also set the standards regarding portion size. Take a look at the shift in the size of portions that consumers have demanded over the past fifty years:

- Fifty years ago, the serving size of a fountain drink was eight ounces.
- Fifty years ago, the hamburger patty was eight to the pound, or two ounces.
- Fifty years ago, the french fries came in a little white bag instead of a large red box.

Are you catching the cultural drift here? Eating a meal back then would be like eating a Happy Meal today and calling it lunch. What was a normal, acceptable portion fifty years ago would be considered a woefully inadequate meal today. Over the years, consumers have demanded larger portions. The skimpy little McDonald's hamburger in a Happy Meal is 250 calories. Now you can get a Double Quarter Pounder with Cheese for almost three times as much, at 740 calories. The french fries in the Happy Meal? For a small fry, you're looking at 250 calories. For grownups, a large serving of fries is more than double that, at 570 calories. What about the drink? A twelve-ounce "child-sized" soda is 110 calories. (You can't even get an eight-ounce drink anymore.) Forget "child-sized!" You can get a thirty-two-ounce drink for a mere 310 calories.

These days, a 610-calorie Happy Meal is only good for kids. It comes in that cute little box with the cute little toy, the cute little hamburger, the cute little bag of fries, and the totally inadequate twelve-ounce drink. You're an adult, so you're going to choose the adult-sized portion at 1,620 calories. (I did not intentionally inflate the numbers. These are right off of the McDonald's official Web site.[6])

I repeat, 1,620 calories. How many calories does your meal-tracking worksheet say you should be consuming per day? I thought so. You eat like this on a regular basis and you're the one who's going to be supersized. And, no, the fault is not with McDonald's. They have simply responded to consumer demand for bigger, better servings over the years. I use them as an example, not to demonize them but as an illustration of how far society has moved off-center in its perception of normal food portions. People have gotten smarter about a lot of things in the past fifty years, but the size of a normal portion isn't one of them. Portions now are based on what people *want* to eat, not what people *should* eat. Portions now are based on *desires*, not on *needs*.

You don't just have this issue with McDonald's; you have it with anything you eat—except maybe brussels sprouts. I remain convinced that any serving size of brussels sprouts is too big. But green, bulbous vegetables aside, because you've grown up in the same society that has demanded bigger portions from McDonald's and other restaurants, you've probably lost a true picture of what a *reasonable* portion is.

Part of your misperception has to do with a high amount of snacking, which I'll talk about in a minute. Snack foods tend to be high in calories, fat, and sodium. So, to make them look "healthier," the food-packaging people (remember the three *p*'s from chapter 3—packaging, processing, and portions?) reduced the size of the portion so all of the calories, fats, and sodium numbers would be smaller. It looks like a great deal until you realize what you normally eat is really five servings, not one.

Generally, in portioning, the higher the caloric content of the food, the smaller the serving size. You want to eat a cup and a half of baby carrots? No problem at around 70 calories. But what about a cup and a half of Ben and Jerry's Heath Bar Crunch ice cream? Well, that's a bit more at 870 calories. The portion size for the carrots is a cup; for Ben and Jerry's, it's half a cup. More calories; smaller serving size.

This is a great rule of thumb. The lower the caloric content of the food (think fruits and vegetables), the more you can eat per serving. Fruits and vegetables are the nutritional "bargain foods." They don't "cost" very much in terms of calories, but they provide an enormous dividend of nutrients, fiber, and fill. That's why your meal-tracking worksheet has you eating a lot of them every day.

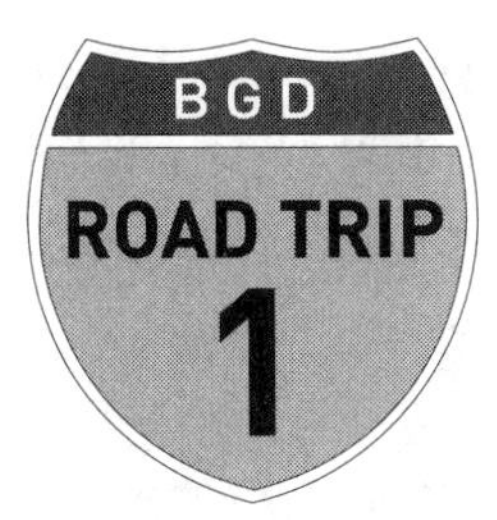

Time to take a break from reading and start confessing. Unlike the people I tend to meet, you're only going to be confessing on paper, not at the T-ball game.

I'd like you to take some time and reflect upon what you discovered in chapter 3 when you went through all of the food in your kitchen and realized what the packaging portion size was. How did you feel about that? Was it surprising to you? Go back and review what you wrote down. (For those of you who failed to truly take advantage of that road trip, it's not too late for you! I invite you to go to your cupboards, your freezer, and your refrigerator to take a look at the portion sizes listed on the packages. I venture to guess that your reaction will be: "They say a serving size is how much?" Unless you're talking about fruits and vegetables, think in ounces, not in cups.)

You've been working through your meal-tracking worksheet and measuring your food in order to calculate your daily and weekly portions. I realize this seems tedious, but it's important for you to work through this information in order to get over the hurdle of ignorant eating. You are becoming informed! You have probably been unaware of the caloric punch of the portions of food you eat. If you ignorantly continue believing the delusion that a cup and a half of Ben and Jerry's is one serving, it's going to be difficult to achieve and maintain the body God designed for you.

Right now, I'd like you to do a little confessing about your portions. Admit that you routinely eat more than you should. This goes back to the concept of accepting yourself. Accept this truth about yourself. Allow this truth to remove the scales from your eyes when it comes to food and how much you eat. Living in denial is only going to add on the pounds year after year. It's said that confession is good for the soul. In this case, confession is good for the body, too.

Once you've confessed, you need to take the next step. It's time to recommit to **(E)—Eating for health**. Health does not allow for gluttony on a regular basis. Gluttony becomes a trap to be avoided. Gluttony is lurking within ignorant eating. Look at this increased knowledge of proper portioning as the best way to avoid the deceptive trap of gluttony.

The Delicate Deception

Do you remember the verse in Proverbs that says, "There is a way that seems right to a man, but in the end it leads to death"? (It's such an important concept that Solomon states it twice—first in Proverbs 14:12 and again in Proverbs 16:25.) Over the past fifty years, society has come to consider a Double Quarter Pounder with Cheese and a large order of fries to be a normal meal. It's a way that seems right. Eating three quarters of a pint of Ben and Jerry's ice cream in one sitting seems right. In actual fact, this is a way that leads to obesity and death. You must consciously veer off this course and return to God's wisdom.

Remember the verse at the beginning of this chapter? What were you warned not to crave? You were warned not to crave "delicacies" because such food is "deceptive." In reality, is the food deceptive? Or have you deceived yourself about the food? It would be nice and easy to just blame the food itself, to brand it evil and bad. The devil made you do it; the Twinkie made you do it; the *delicacies* made you do it. In truth, food is amoral; it is what it is. If there's deception going on, it's not coming from the food. You're the one deceiving yourself about eating those delicacies.

What do you think of when you hear the word *delicacies*? I think of those frosting-covered little petit fours you often see around the holidays. You just know by looking at them that they're going to be really good, really caloric, and really hard to resist. I certainly think these types of food can give you trouble, as the Proverbs verse says. A delicacy is defined as something that is pleasing to eat and considered rare or luxurious. Because people tend to save them for the holidays, those little squares, along with fudge and Christmas cookies, do send up an irresistible siren song.

But I think you can get in trouble with the opposite kind of food, too, which happens pretty much year-round. I think you can get in trouble with food that's still pleasing to eat but is hardly rare and rarely luxurious. I'm talking about your ubiquitous snack food. This brings me to the second hurdle you must overcome to achieve the body God designed for you: mindless eating, or autopilot eating.

Let's go back to the baby boomer thing. (Even if you aren't a baby boomer, you're probably influenced by us because we've been the engine of change in this country for the past several decades.) One trend that has really taken off in my generation is snacking. Of course, Generation Xers (born between 1960 and 1980) and Millennials (born between 1980 and 2000) have perfected snacking in conjunction with computer use. (Think of Sandra Bullock in the first part of the movie *The Net* living on pizza and chips while seated in front of her computer.) But I think my generation needs to take ownership of the beginning of this trend. Why? Because baby boomers are also known as the television generation, being the first generation of Americans born into the glorious milieu of broadcast media.

When I think of autopilot eating, I automatically think of television. What happens when you sit down in front of the television with a bag of chips or pretzels or cookies? You're sitting there, enjoying the show, munching away. Before you know it, you've eaten the entire bag of whatever. Now, you probably were a little bit hungry when you reached for the bag (we'll talk about the other possibility in the next chapter). If you were really hungry, you would have eaten a meal. But you were a little bit hungry, so you grabbed something quick to snack on while you watched television. Just sitting there, not really hungry, you've just eaten three ounces of corn chips at 450 calories or three ounces of pretzels at 300 calories or three cookies at almost 500 calories. All that on autopilot, without really thinking about it or really paying much attention to what you were eating. It's your mouth moving and you swallowing, all while concentrating on the latest episode of *Law and Order*, and now 300 to 500 calories out of your day are gone, used up, finito. If you have around a 2,000-calorie allotment per day, you've just mindlessly consumed a fourth of your day's calories without getting very much in return—and frankly, without really paying much attention. It's not like you even enjoyed those cookies; they existed merely as a culinary form of *white noise* to your preoccupation with the show.

That's why I say that today's "delicacies" include snack foods such as tortilla chips and pretzels and cookies. They're foods you crave, and they're deceptive. When you're eating them, it seems like you're not really eating much of anything, but their calories, fat, and sodium make a big impact on your overall diet.

They're deceptive in another way—they give the appearance of nutrition without any of the substance of nutrition. They are satisfying.

They fill you up, but they provide very little of the components you need to function properly. This doesn't mean I'm saying *death to all snack food forever*; I'm talking about putting these foods into proper context. For example, I like SunChips. A serving is an ounce, which figures out to be roughly twelve chips at 140 calories. It would not be a problem for me to eat a serving of SunChips with a healthy sandwich for lunch. The problem comes when I grab the bag of SunChips in the evening after eating dinner and go through three servings (420 calories) without really thinking about it.

I don't know what your favorite snack foods are, but it's time to take another road trip to your kitchen to find out.

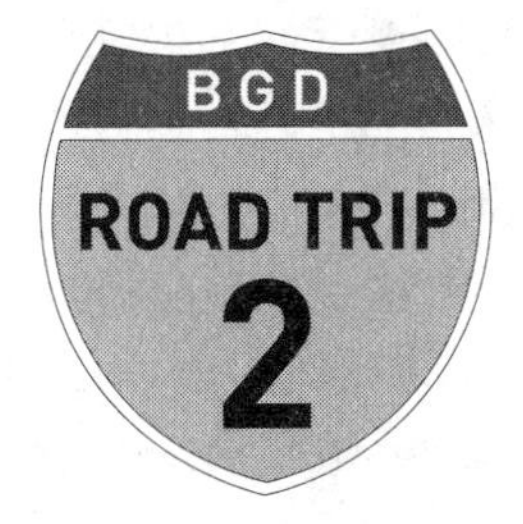

This time I want you to return to the kitchen and write down what your autopilot or mindless foods are. Look in your cabinets, freezer, and fridge. My autopilot food may be SunChips, but yours is probably something completely different. If you're having trouble confessing to yourself what those are, just think of your weekly trip to the grocery store. You may not have much memory of actually eating that bag of pretzels, but it will show up in your grocery cart.

Speaking of your groceries, what items are routinely on your grocery list? You may *say* you're eating this or that, but the tale is told by the list. What you buy is really what you eat. What will you leave your house for at 10:00 at night, in the rain, to go get at the store? OK, got it? Now, write it down. It will be good for you to see it in print. It cannot hurt you on paper, but your habit of eating it can. Put it down, name it, and you have already weakened its power over you. You are rejecting mindlessness and reengaging your brain.

Put yourself mentally in your car, driving home from work. What do you think about eating when you get home? This is before you actually eat dinner. What do you snack on just to "tide you over"? Go ahead and write it down. I want you to be aware of what you're reaching for and when.

And since we're on mindless eating, what about at work or in your car? Mindless eating doesn't just happen in front of a television or a computer. It happens anytime your focus is on something else while you eat. Expand your definition and write down what, when, and how often you engage in autopilot eating.

Next, given some of the calorie counts I used as examples in this chapter, guesstimate how much you're consuming while mindlessly eating. If you really want to be specific about it because you think that surely it can't be as much as you've guessed, then get out your food book or go to an online calorie counter for help.[7] Calculate how many calories this type of eating tallies up for you each day, each week, each month. Remembering that 3,500 calories is a pound of body fat, what are we really talking about here? If I eat my SunChips on autopilot three days a week, that's 1,260 calories per week, or 5,460 calories per month, or over one and a half pounds of body fat per month in SunChips alone! I like them, but I don't like them that much!

My hope is that once you've done this, you'll recognize the existence of these mindless calories. The goal is for you to be deceived by this food no longer. Just because this food is easy to eat and easy to forget doesn't mean it does not have an impact on your health and the body God designed for you.

Discretion, Not Deception

The calories you are supposed to eat each day have a God-given purpose. Their purpose is to fuel your body to allow you to carry out God's will. First Corinthians 6:19 clearly says that your body doesn't belong to you; it is the temple of God's Holy Spirit. Paul puts it this way in Galatians 2:20, "I have been crucified with Christ and I no longer live, but Christ lives in me. The life I live in the body, I live by faith in the Son of God, who loved me and gave himself for me." It isn't about you and what you want to eat, ignorantly, mindlessly, or otherwise. It's about a body that belongs to God, a flesh-and-bone temple for God's Spirit. When you squander those caloric resources, which were meant for a nutritional purpose by God, you act in a way contrary to His will.

Does this mean that God is only happy when I eat bean sprouts and tofu? Not if by eating bean sprouts and tofu I'm trying to attain some sort of righteousness or perfection in my own eyes. Romans 10:2–3 speaks of those with this attitude: "For I can testify about them that they are zealous for God, but their zeal is not based on knowledge. Since they did not know the righteousness that comes from God and sought to establish their own, they did not submit to God's righteousness." The danger here is to believe that somehow eating bean sprouts (notice I didn't—wouldn't ever—say brussels sprouts) and tofu somehow makes you righteous. Righteousness comes from God, not the foods we eat.

When you eat in a healthful way, you are benefiting your body and honoring the God who created it at the same time. You are saying, "I submit to Your design, Lord, and I choose to eat the foods and the amounts that will contribute to, not detract from, my body's health."

I'm not suggesting that the goal here is persistent navel-gazing and restriction where food is concerned. After all, Jesus is quite clear in the Gospels that life is more important than food (Matthew 6:25; Luke 12:23). Food is to enhance your life, not to rule it.

You have been given a certain amount of "discretionary spending" in your nutrition bank. God has given you an absolute abundance of choices, which include sweets and what the meal-tracking worksheet calls "discretionary" choices. These discretionary calories equal about 15 percent of the total daily amount of calories you are to consume, including fats and sweets. Naturally, to live a healthy life, you need to limit these foods in your overall diet. But there's nothing that says you must eliminate them completely. You have the freedom to make choices. You run into trouble when you consider *all* of your calories discretionary. That is a deception.

Do you remember the concept earlier of end-user modifications versus original equipment? Allowing too many foods to become part of your discretionary eating brings about end-user modifications in the form of excess weight and degraded health. However, when you eat in a healthy manner, you show your submission to God's original equipment and to His will.

In this chapter I've talked about two hurdles: (1) ignorant eating, especially when it comes to the portions you really need, and (2) mindless, autopilot eating. These are two areas where it is possible to make immediate, quantifiable changes in your habits in order to consume fewer calories each day and thereby lose weight. You've been reminded that healthy eating does not produce righteousness and that your life is more than food.

You are told to love the Lord with all your heart, soul, mind, and strength (Mark 12:30; Luke 10:27). Think about that third component as it relates to what I've talked about in this chapter. You're to love God with your mind. That means you are to love the things of God with your mind. Your body is a gift from God; it is the living temple of His Holy Spirit on this earth. Therefore, you are to love your body with your mind. No more ignorant eating! No more mindless eating! You must be informed and intentional about what you eat, how much you eat, and when you eat. You have no more excuses. Once you know the truth of something, you become responsible to respond to that truth.

Eating God's way will bring you vitality and the freedom of good health. It will save you from the trap of gluttony and all its companion miseries. It is not the same as the freedom to eat whatever you want, because that results in enslavement to food, to gluttony, to excess weight. Freedom comes when you honor God. Freedom is the ability to eat a single cookie without guilt and be satisfied.

> *Father, I confess I have been eating without thinking, desiring to just fill my belly without a thought to how this affects my health. I commit myself to intentionally thinking about every bite of food I put in my mouth. Mindless eating is such an ingrained habit, Lord. I confess I will need Your help to overcome it. When I falter, bring the truth of Your plan for my health to mind. Help me to see food in its proper context, as fuel from You, as a blessing from You to be used for the good of my body, and not for the indulgence of my will. May Your*

will be done in my eating, Father, not mine. Be with me in this. Give me strength to do what is right. I thank You in advance for Your forgiveness when I fall. Pick me back up, and set me on the right path to health. I trust that my life in You is more than food. Be with me as I commit these things to You. Amen.

Chapter 8

Midnight at the Kitchen Oasis

But woe to you who are rich, for you have already received your comfort.

—Luke 6:24

We live in a rich, blessed country. We are able to find comfort in a variety of ways. One of the ways we choose to seek comfort is through the panacea of pastries. But could it be that God wants us to turn to Him for comfort instead? Prayer or potato chips? Meditation or munchies? Deity or doughnuts?

In the last chapter, we tackled the concepts of ignorant and mindless eating. I concluded by discussing the choice to eat for health. That sounds so simple, doesn't it? It's like the commercial says, "Just do it." Eat for health. Given the statistic that almost 80 percent of us aren't taking Nike's advice and "just doing it" where exercise is concerned, is it any wonder that a Nike approach to healthy eating is equally ineffective? Eating for health isn't that simple for most of us. Something is getting in the way of our "just doing it." Once you've tackled ignorant and mindless eating, there's still a huge factor to be considered. It's the eight-hundred-pound gorilla in the room of healthy eating, and it's called comfort eating. It's time to take it on.

The Warm Embrace of Comfort Food

Few things bring as much comfort as homemade bread, especially when it's hot out of the oven and slathered with sweet cream butter. It's warm; it's soft; it's delicious. I went to a charity event recently, and one of the items up for bid in the silent auction part was called Delivered Comfort—homemade bread delivered to your house every week for two months. It was a very popular item. People would walk along the tables, reading all of the cards and descriptions of items to bid on, and when they'd come to this one, there was almost a universal sigh. "Oh, fresh hot bread every week!" You could hear the longing in their voices.

This was the sort of silent auction where everyone has a bidder number and a certain amount of time to mark their bids on a sheet of paper. (If you haven't experienced this kind of genteel warfare, I encourage you to attend a charity auction. As a therapist, I find them fascinating. You can view an interesting variety of bad behavior, all for a good cause.)

Anyway, back to the bread. I kept track of this item because it intrigued me more than the crocheted potholders, restaurant coupons, and beauty salon certificates. Watching this particular bid sheet, I kept seeing the same bidder number. As other bidders outbid her, this bidder kept upping the ante. Finally, the bidder must have thought, "To heck with it!" and signed up for the "guaranteed bid," which meant she would pay any higher price, thus guaranteeing herself the winning bid. It was her way of saying, "Back off, Jack! The bread is mine!"

Aren't you like that about your comfort food? You tend to get grouchy if anyone tries to interfere with it. You *need* that food. It's your reward. It helps you feel good. You use it to cope. It brings you back to your happy place. It's your comfort.

In an increasingly uncomfortable world, comfort food takes on new importance. You've dealt with ignorant and mindless eating, but comfort food isn't ignorant or mindless. You know precisely what you're after when you eat it and give it your complete and undivided attention. You don't just eat it; you *revel* in it.

It is no accident that comfort food tends to be high in carbohydrates from grains and sugar. You're after a certain outcome where this food is concerned, and without really knowing the science of it, you stumbled upon starchy, sugary foods to achieve that feeling. Your unscientific trial and error with the pantry produces a very scientific result. Foods high in carbohydrates cause your body to have an increased supply of a substance called *serotonin*. Serotonin is a neurotransmitter, which is a fancy way of saying it provides a pathway for nerves to talk to each other. When your nerves are communicating with each other through serotonin, you feel relaxed and calm. If you have a lot of serotonin, you can feel drowsy. After that really big pasta meal on Sunday afternoon, what do you want to do? Why, take a nap! That's serotonin at work.

One of the precursors of serotonin is tryptophan. If your body has tryptophan, it can make serotonin. Do you know what has a large amount of tryptophan? Turkey. After a big Thanksgiving meal, you sigh, stretch, feel extremely content, then curl up on the sofa and snooze. This is your body on tryptophan.

Comfort food is physical, and it is emotional. It is snuggly, cuddly, feel-good food. The world can be harsh, stark, and edgy, so it's no surprise that you like your feel-good food. It's no surprise you can get pretty militant about it. Even if you're increasing your fruits and vegetables each day, this type of food can be difficult to give up, because if you give it up, you think you're giving up comfort itself.

It's not enough to add fruits and vegetables to your diet. It's not enough to give up snacking. You need to come clean about your comfort food.

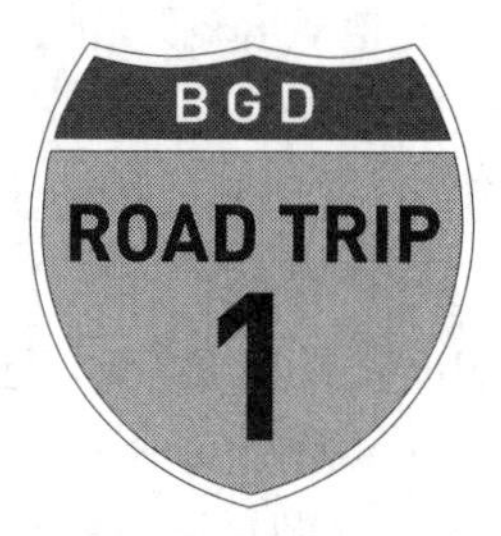

This isn't really a full-blown BGD Road Trip; it's more like a BGD Side Trip. I want you to take a minute and write a list of your comfort foods. Now, this certainly could include the kind of snack foods I talked about before, but your list probably needs to be expanded. Comfort food is the type of "normal" food you tend to overeat. It could be bread, rolls, desserts, or mashed potatoes with lots of butter or sour cream. Don't just think about your habits between meals; think about what you eat *at* meals.

Remember when your mother told you that you couldn't have dessert until you ate all of your vegetables? This normal mom behavior was a bit of a set-up, actually, because it made vegetables something to be endured on your way to the really good stuff. How many of you would chew your vegetables as quick as you could and take a huge swig of milk to wash down the offending mouthful? What made that torture palatable was the thought of the chocolate cake at the end of the meal. Bingo! Vegetables as torture. Dessert as reward.

You're an adult now, and you no longer look to your mom to tell you what to eat. Right? Well, just think about that for a minute. What foods do you "endure" in order to eat what you really want? What foods do you tend to linger over to allow to blossom in all your senses so you can enjoy every nuance, every tactile experience? What foods do you tend to inhale, as if you just can't seem to get enough of them (and if you could lie down in a bathtub and absorb these foods through your skin, you would)? Write them down. These are the foods you've just self-disclosed as your comfort foods. You need to watch what they are because your relationship with these foods has to change. God designed your body to be a temple of God, and if there's one thing God won't tolerate, it's competition.

The Seven Deadly Sins

Let's review the seven deadly sins I talked about earlier. These are like the seven dwarves of excess (Hi ho! Hi ho! It's off to greed we go!) Unlike Walt Disney's seven dwarves (Sleepy, Sneezy, Happy, Grumpy, Bashful, Dopey, and Doc—there, I gave them to you so you won't stop everything until you can name all seven), the seven deadly sins have names like Pride, Greed, Lust, Envy, Anger, Slothfulness, and Gluttony. In general, each of these seven takes a normal reaction and carries it to excess:

- Pride: There's nothing wrong with being proud of your accomplishments, but Scripture clearly says you are to boast only in the Lord (Galatians 6:14). If you get too full of yourself, the pleasure you gain for a job well done turns to pride.

- Greed: Money, in and of itself, is not wrong. Neither is wealth. But an excessive love of money is, and it's called greed. Greed is condemned in Mark 7:21–23, along with a pretty disgusting list of evil thoughts that make a person unclean. Greed may be culturally acceptable, but it is spiritually gross.
- Lust: Lust takes the normal, God-given attraction for members of the opposite sex, which was all part of His plan for marriage (read Song of Solomon if you have doubts about that), and steers it into self-absorbed overdrive. Jesus specifically warns against lust in Matthew 5:28.
- Envy: Competition is a natural reaction, and it can be good. Hebrews 10:24 urges us to outdo each other in love and good deeds. But if you're like me, you sometimes don't know when to stop being competitive and end up in Galatians 5:26, boastful about yourself and living in envy of others.
- Anger: Anger is also natural; it's hardwired into your mind and body. Scripture (Ephesians 4:26) says that it's possible to be angry within God's boundaries. People, however, lose all sense of proportion as James 1:20 says. You may express righteous indignation in your anger; however, for most people, anger is anything but righteous.
- Slothfulness: That's just a great word. Of course, it doesn't appear at all in the New International Version or the New American Standard Version of the Bible. Go to the King James Version, however, and there's a whole lotta slothfulness goin' on in Proverbs. It

means laziness. (My favorite verse about slothfulness is Proverbs 26:14: "As the door turneth upon his hinges, so doth the slothful upon his bed" [KJV].) Now, there's nothing wrong with resting. God set apart His Sabbath as a day of rest, which is good. He knew you would need downtime. However, perpetual downtime is excessive and slothful.

- Gluttony: Finally, I arrive at gluttony (and yes, I've also arrived at my point). Gluttony takes the natural pleasure God designed into the act of eating and uses it for excessive self-gratification. Comfort food is not an inaccurate nom de plume for your overeating. If eating this food wasn't gratifying in some way, you wouldn't do it to excess.

Idol Eating, Not *Idle* Eating

With comfort food, eating food for food's sake isn't your problem. Your problem is your relationship with your food. Your food is lover, friend, and comforter. When this happens, food becomes a God substitute, or to put it another way, food becomes an *idol*. Back in the Old Testament, God warned the people of Israel over and over again not to worship idols of wood and stone. In most Christian households today, I would venture to guess there aren't too many wood or stone idols hanging around, but I wouldn't be so sure about ones made out of carbohydrates.

Worshiping wood and stone idols has always been pointless and ineffective. In fact, it seems a little bizarre that, after seeing all of God's bona fide miracles on the way out of Egypt, Aaron and the people of Israel thought making a golden calf was a good idea. What were they thinking? The people themselves provided the gold for the calf, and they watched it being molded, so how could they possibly think it contained some sort of divine power? They weren't divine, so how could something they made be divine? You may read about what they did and dismiss their foolishness. You might be right there with God in Isaiah 2:8 as you shake your head and smugly declare, "How ridiculous! What were they thinking?"

But haven't you done the same thing with your comfort food? You either buy or make this food that gives you comfort as if it has some sort of power greater than its ingredients. You give it that power by declaring it has that power, just as the people of Israel declared that the calf they had made would substitute for God. You end up scooping yourself a bowl of ice cream and then worshiping it because it is somehow going to solve your problems or salve your wounds. You worship the loaf of banana bread because, by eating it, you're going to magically forget the stress of the day. You worship the chocolate chip cookies because eating them is a transcendent experience that harkens back to Mom's kitchen and simpler days when someone else took care of you.

This all has to do with your relationship with food; it has nothing to do with nutrition. It puts you outside the bounds of God's will for the body He designed.

Food as Lover

Food has a profound effect on the body. It's not unlike a drug or alcohol. It is not mere coincidence that gluttony is often linked to drunkenness. Both are excessive and demonstrate a lack of self-control. But there's more going on than just saying no. When food is your lover, friend, and comforter, it's a relationship that's very difficult to give up. It becomes a relationship that defines your life.

I remember when I first fell in love with my wife, LaFon. It was back in college. She was absolutely amazing, a dynamo of optimism and energy (and she still is). She made me feel like there wasn't anything I couldn't do or accomplish. I felt so good being around her that I wanted to be with her all the time. When I couldn't see her, I called her on the phone. (This was, of course, back in the old days before cell phones when you had to actually *wait* for someone to be near a phone! How did we manage?) We talked for hours. I could not—and cannot—imagine my life without her. She defines who I am as a person. God wasn't kidding when He talked about cleaving in Genesis 2:24. We have truly become one flesh, and we both would say that it's difficult to tell where one of us stops and the other begins.

I've just shared with you the wonder and gratitude that embodies my relationship with my wife. Sadly, I have had people sit in my office and describe that same relationship but with food. Food is all they think about. They cannot imagine life without their comfort food. Food and its effects define who they are as a person. It's difficult for them to identify where their personality stops and their relationship with food begins. Food is their lover just as LaFon is my wife.

In a loving marriage relationship, you have trust because you know that person has your own best interests at heart. The relationship is two sided; there is a give and a take. Food, however, is a one-sided relationship. No matter how much you may worship its comforting effects, it cares nothing for you. You can cry out as hard and as loud as those four hundred fifty prophets of Baal in 1 Kings 18:16–40, but food is never going to give you your heart's desire. It's incapable of doing so. To allow anything to have that kind of power over you is dangerous and detrimental. You have given it the power it has, and you already know that your own power is not sufficient to take care of your problems. Only one other can be truly sufficient for you—God (2 Corinthians 12:9).

It's time to leave your lover. I understand how difficult this is because of the emotional investment you've made in food. But remember, this is an attachment you yourself have woven. Since you wove it, you can unravel it. If you've taken your Hershey's bars and your Nestle chocolate chips and formed a chocolate "calf" (much like the golden calf that Aaron and the people of Israel fashioned while Moses was away receiving the Ten Commandments), it's time to admit it and repent. If you've taken your doughnuts and your desserts and bowed down before the altar of sweets, it's time to admit it and repent. If you've taken your breads and your baked goods and infused them with magical powers, it's time to admit it and repent.

It's not as if God is unaware of your idolatry. When Moses was up on Sinai communing with God and getting the Ten Commandments, he didn't know what was happening at the base of the mountain. But God did. He had to interrupt His time with Moses to have him skedaddle back down the mountain because of the foolishness of Aaron and others (Exodus 32:7). God knows what's in your heart and how you're using food. He wants you to turn from your lover, your self-created idol, and return to Him.

God wants to be your source of companionship, friendship, comfort, and love through your worship of and relationship with Him. Your life is to be all about Him, not all about food. The pleasure He designed into food was meant to be a gift, not a substitute for Him. When you substitute something else for Him, you make God jealous because of your unfaithfulness and grieved because He knows the ultimate outcome of your choices.

This brings me back to the seven dwarves of excess, the seven deadly sins. You can end up using each of these as a way to gain affirmation, worthiness, acceptance, security, love, power, and comfort to meet your emotional needs. But doing so leads you to sin and away from God.

- Instead of believing God's affirmation of your worth, you can become prideful about your own accomplishments.
- Instead of trusting in God's provision for your life, you can become greedy for material wealth.
- Instead of honoring God's plan for sex, you can lust after others.
- Instead of enjoying contentment found in God, you can envy your brothers.
- Instead of seeking God's peace, you can live in a state of anger or fear.
- Instead of pursuing God's purpose, you can waste your life in slothfulness.
- Instead of being satisfied with God's comfort, you can fill yourself with food.

Fifty Ways to Leave Your Lover

This isn't a pretty picture, but it's an honest one. Do you remember the verse that started off this chapter? "But woe to you who are rich, for you have already received your comfort" (Luke 6:24). That's such a sad commentary about those who are content with the mere benefits of this world, trading them in for the vast rewards of heaven. It's kind of like a small child who is so enamored with the bow on the package that he has no interest in the amazing gift inside.

When you substitute other things, including food, for God, you keep the tiny little bow and throw out the wondrous gift in the package. Is there comfort to be received in this life? Absolutely. The verse in Luke says so. However, it's a faint shadow of what awaits you. When you exchange the worldly for the divine, you settle for so much less. Jesus warns in several places (see the sixth chapter of Matthew) that it is quite possible for you to receive your reward in full in the here and now through your behavior, thus forfeiting the future blessings that could have come.

That's why I say it's time to leave your worldly lover and reclaim your heavenly relationship. If it comes down to prayer or potato chips, choose prayer. If it comes down to meditation or munchies, choose meditation. If it comes down to deity or doughnuts, choose deity. As the song says, there must be fifty ways to leave your lover.

Timing Is Everything

Before you take off on your next road trip, let's talk about the timing of your comfort food. It's important to be aware of what your comfort foods are, but you also need to be aware of when you meet your food lover. It may be a morning rendezvous with a sugary pastry and a large cup of flavored coffee. It may be in the car on the way home with a bag of cookies or chocolate. It may be at home at night in your easy chair with a bowl of ice cream. It may be a bag of chips before dinner. It may be finishing off that pie or cake after everyone else has gone to bed.

Be aware that just as an adulterous relationship has a pattern of trysts, there may be a time and a place you've set aside for your comfort foods. In some ways, just putting yourself in that time or place can trigger your desire for those foods, even if that wasn't your original intent. You've created a pattern, and your body responds to it.

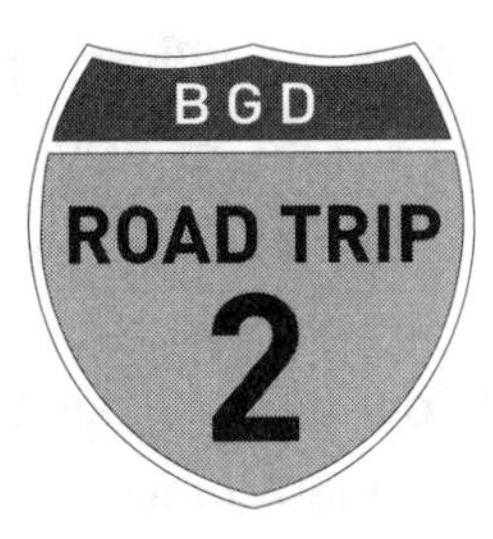

It's time to get out your Bible and turn to 1 Kings 18:16–40. I want you to read about Elijah and the prophets of Baal and Asherah and think about how you've turned the comfort food in your life into an idol. How many times, like those prophets, have you turned to food to produce results in your life, only to be disappointed and humiliated? How many times have you danced around your food of comfort, giving it your time and energy, only to be left feeling empty and unsatisfied at the response?

God wants you to trust Him as Elijah did. He wants to be given the opportunity to prove to you, as He proved to the people of Israel, that He alone is God and that He is sufficient for your needs.

What idol will you offer to God for this demonstration? You've already written down your foods of comfort; now I want you to add your times of comfort. For the next week, I want you to identify these foods and times as ones you are going to intentionally give up to God. If it is *imperative* you start your day with a venti caramel frappuccino and a pumpkin loaf at Starbucks, recognize this as a false god. The outcome of your day is not dependent upon consuming these items. They have no power over your day besides what you give them. If you decide the day only goes well when you have them, you sabotage the day if you don't. They're inanimate objects! They are wood and stone!

They are made with hands and fingers by people who are as powerless as you are to dictate the way your day will turn out.

So identify your idol, and then call in your spiritual reinforcements. Instead of your breakfast at Starbucks, eat at home, and use the time to read your Bible or talk to your family. As you drive past the drive-through, pray for strength and resolve. Meditate not on what you're missing but on what you've gained through your authentic relationship with God. Say to yourself, "I am Elijah, not a prophet of Baal. I will trust in God to validate me, not in a false idol. This day belongs to God, not to food."

Write down each and every idol because almost all of us have more than one. Idols don't just come in singles, so don't be surprised if you have several to weed out of your life. Take them on one at a time. Victory in one will help motivate you to take on another.

On your meal-tracking worksheet, I want you to use the bottom to record your victories each day over your comfort food idols. Call it "Idol Victories," and add a couple of exclamation points. Remember, it's not enough to just eat your fruits and vegetables along with all of your comfort food. Slowly, over time, through baby steps, give up these other food relationships. I promise that God is ready, willing, and able to be a much better friend, companion, and comforter than whatever it is you're eating. His love for you is genuine and not dependent upon the short-lived punch of your neurotransmitters.

We've talked in this chapter about comfort and love and lovers. The church is called the bride of Christ. God has always had a lover's heart for His people. Listen to what God says to you through Solomon in that great book on love: "Place me like a seal over your heart, like a seal on your arm; for love is as strong as death, its jealousy unyielding as the grave. It burns like blazing fire, like a mighty flame" (Song of Solomon 8:6). In the story of Elijah, God's fire burned like a mighty flame and gave witness to His power and presence. Allow God's love to do the same in your own life.

> *Father, I confess my idolatry. I have used food as a false god to provide me with comfort, companionship, and love. I did not turn to You for these things but turned instead to those things I could control, those things I could obtain for myself. I did not trust You to provide what I needed. Forgive me, Father. Help me to lay these comfort foods on Your altar. Consume them and remove the power I have given over to them. Help me to see my unfaithfulness to You in the choices I have made with food. Return to me the joy of Your love, comfort, and companionship. Return food to its proper place in my life. I thank You for the pleasure You designed into food and ask for Your help in placing it into proper perspective. May each day bring me closer to leaning on You to provide for my emotional needs. May I turn to food when I'm hungry but to You when I'm sad or depressed or lonely or anxious. May I turn to food when I'm hungry but to You when I'm tired or bored or distracted or frustrated. May I turn to food when I'm hungry but to You when I'm fearful or worried or angry or joyful. May I turn to food when my body is truly hungry but to You when it's my soul that hungers. Help me, God, to recognize the difference. Amen.*

Chapter 9

Be Still and Know That I Am Chocolate

Be still, and know that I am God.

—Psalm 46:10

One of the biggest causes of unnecessary weight gain in this country is stress. It affects what we choose to eat and how our bodies react to what we eat. For the person wanting to gain health and lose weight, it is vital to slow down long enough to realize you need to slow down.

In the last chapter, I talked about your relationship with food as idolatry, and I talked about how the Israelites sinned at the foot of Mount Sinai when Aaron led them in crafting a golden calf to worship. Think about that story a little bit more as you consider the role stress plays in your life. I think it will be instructive; you can learn more about how ordinary things in your life today can be transformed into idols.

I Can't Be Still!

In order to make this comparison, get out your Bible and turn to Exodus 32. Moses has been up on Mount Sinai communing with God and receiving the Law. (If you've ever read through Exodus and perhaps Leviticus, you'll know why he was up on that mountain for a while. Every time I'm tempted to skim through these parts of Scripture, I have to remember that if God took the time to say all of this to a human being, then this human being can at least take the time to read it.) So, at the beginning of Exodus 32, the people are getting antsy. They don't really know how long it's supposed to take or really what Moses is doing up there; they've just been told to camp out and wait. Or, to put it another way, they've just been told to *be still.* That's where they run into problems.

The people decide it is taking too long, even though they have no idea how long it's supposed to take. They decide Moses has delayed coming down. It can be pretty irritating when someone else delays you. The other person doesn't seem to be respecting your time or your priorities. They're saying their agenda is more important than yours. How dare they! Think of the irritation you feel when someone delays you ten seconds while you're driving to work or a minute and a half in a line at a store. Imagine the irritation the people of Israel felt after being left to twiddle their thumbs for over a month.

Because Moses is "delayed," they're ready to turn his God in for something a little bit more reliable. They ask Aaron to make for them a god who can go before them since Moses is apparently MIA (missing in action). They're tired of being still; they're stressed out from waiting for Moses and not knowing what in the world is going to happen. In order to alleviate that stress, they decide it's time to take action, to create a substitute god and "to eat and to drink, and... to play" (Exodus 32:6, NASU).

That was then. Let's fast-forward into the here and now. The Israelites were anxious about Moses being gone for so long and not confident of what the future would bring, so they made themselves a golden calf. We are anxious over any number of things and not confident of what the future will bring, so we resort to chocolate or our other comfort foods. To quell all anxious fears, past and present, God softly whispers the words of Psalm 46:10: "Be still, and know that I am God."

The Stress Equation

Please don't think I'm minimizing stress. This is a huge factor in our lives, for we live in a pretty stressful time. (Can I hear an "amen" to that?) At least, we've *decided* we live in a pretty stressful time. I'm not sure wandering around a wilderness, being chased by hostile forces, encountering thirst and hunger, even experiencing the mighty miracles of God are any less stressful than what I encounter in my day-to-day life. Come to think of it, I'm not sure the stresses I face are really as big as the stresses the Israelites faced—slavery, freedom, escape, pursuit, miracles, enemies, death and destruction, deliverance, desert, etc. Perhaps our stress has more to do with perception than reality. Perhaps part of the stress equation is what we *decide* is stressful.

How do you spell S-T-R-E-S-S?

I work with people's problems pretty much all day. People will often come up to me in other settings and say, "I couldn't do what you do!" To them, being around and being involved in the problems of others is far too stressful; they just couldn't be a therapist or counselor. Now, in our branches, we have people who work on the office side of things—not clinical but clerical—handling the day-to-day operations. More than once, I've heard counselors tell one of our office people, "I couldn't do what you do!" To them, being around phones and paperwork and financial details is far too stressful; they just couldn't work in an office.

You decide what is stressful in your life. The fewer things you decide are stressful, the calmer you are. This turns out to be harder than it sounds in the real world. Stress is a part of life. It is a physical and emotional reaction to any change in status, which means you're under some level of stress from the moment you wake to when you fall asleep. Just as you found that *fat* wasn't necessarily a bad word, *stress* isn't either. It all depends upon the type of stress and your response to it.[1]

Acute and chronic stress

Acute stress is the slam-on-the-brakes kind of stress. It's tied to a specific event that is perceived as either dangerous or demanding. Your body rallies around the emotional reaction of alarm and fear by preparing itself for fight or flight. In fact, that's what the physical reaction is called: "the fight or flight response." When confronted with a dangerous or demanding situation, you're either going to run away like crazy or put up your dukes and fight.

Acute stress and your body's reaction to it can be very beneficial. If I'm the person who has just mindlessly stepped out in front of your car, I want you to experience the slam-on-the-brakes kind of stress! If you don't, I'm in trouble. There are simply times in your life when dangerous or demanding situations arise and must be dealt with for your own safety and for the safety of others.

When acute stress occurs, your heart beats faster and your breathing speeds up because your body produces adrenaline. You're pumped! In the heat of the moment, all of that extra energy and heightened physical response may be necessary if you need to fight your way out of a problem or run away from it. The body, of course, does not judge between a true *fight or flight* situation and a false alarm or close call. Once the immediate danger has passed, your body calms down and returns to normal.

Although the situation may be resolved fairly quickly, acute stress can have lingering effects. Your heart and breathing return to normal, but you may have trouble concentrating for several hours or longer after the event. Muscles that tensed and became taut during the incident may be sore for a while. You may feel a bit queasy or have an unsettled stomach. These symptoms tend to go away eventually.

Chronic stress is the drawn-out-over-time type of stress. It's the water drops dripping on your head. Just one drop isn't a problem, but if that drip continues drop after drop, day after day, month after month, year after year, it builds up and makes you hypersensitive to that next little plop! At that next little plop, you go ballistic and yell out, "That's it! I can't take it anymore!" Others, who are unaware of the dripping, look at you askew and think, "Whew! What's wrong with that guy?" This is a state people find themselves in when faced with difficult, ongoing situations such as an unhappy home life or stressful job. There's no slam-on-the-brakes emergency but a continual drip-drip-drip of a demanding situation that never seems to go away.

Chronic stress has some pretty significant health impacts. When your life is filled with ongoing stress, it takes a toll. Here is a list of stress symptoms from WebMD:[2]

- Rapid heartbeat
- Headache
- Stiff neck and/or tight shoulders
- Backache
- Rapid breathing

- Sweating and sweaty palms
- Upset stomach, nausea, or diarrhea
- Feeling irritated or frustrated at even minor disturbances, losing your temper more often, and yelling at others for no reason
- Feeling jumpy and exhausted all the time
- Finding it hard to concentrate or focus on tasks
- Worrying too much about insignificant things
- Doubting your ability to do things
- Imagining negative, terrifying, or worrisome scenes
- Feeling you are missing opportunities because you can't act quickly

The effects of chronic stress, as you can see, are pretty debilitating. They include both physical and psychological effects. It's no wonder you turn to food to return to your happy place when you have come under an onslaught of these types of symptoms. Of course, while it provides you with a temporary distraction, all of that food does nothing in the long run except add more stress to your life as you stress out about your weight.

The Sky Is Falling! The Sky Is Falling!

I am willing to concede that the people of Israel were experiencing some stress at the base of Mount Sinai. They were living through awesome and amazing times, times both dangerous and demanding. The flight from Egypt and the journey to the Promised Land were not accomplished overnight. They needed to adjust to an ongoing, demanding situation. Quite clearly, they were experiencing the effects of stress by beginning to doubt their ability to do things (or certainly Moses's ability to do things) and imagining negative, terrifying, or worrisome scenes. With Moses still up on the mountain, the people of Israel felt they were missing out on opportunities and needed to take action—which are signs of stress.

What started out as a pretty understandable reaction turned into open rebellion. What would cause the people of Israel to openly rebel and disobey God? I believe one reason is they interpreted their situation as a *crisis*. In crises, the rules often don't apply or get cast aside in the heat of the moment. Theirs wasn't a true crisis, but neither are many of our stressful situations. Some of us turn our own stress into crises so the regular rules don't apply. You know how it goes: "If I'm in a crisis of stress, I can eat that Krispy Kreme because it's the only thing I know will make me feel better. And it's a crisis, so the regular rules and my meal-tracking worksheet won't apply."

I think it's time to redefine *crisis* so you can help yourself redefine *stress*.

Do you remember the children's story *Chicken Little*? It was made into an animated movie, but I'd like you to think back to the original story. In that story, Chicken Little is out and about one day when an acorn falls on her head. She immediately assumes that the sky is falling and reacts in sheer panic. Along her way to inform the king of this crisis, she meets Henny Penny, Ducky Lucky, Goosey Loosey, and Turkey Lurkey. (Try saying those names five times fast.) All of these fowl friends buy right into the crisis that the sky is falling and run pell-mell to find the king. Oh, there's one more character—Foxy Loxy, who, upon hearing of the crisis, offers to escort them all to see the king. He, as the end of the story goes, delivers them promptly to his own den and not to the king, where they encounter a real-life crisis and are never heard from again.

There are many morals to this story, but the one I want to emphasize is at the beginning. Chicken Little took an ordinary event and turned it into a crisis. Acorns grow on oak trees and are meant to fall to the ground. Otherwise, there wouldn't be more oak trees. So falling acorns is not a crisis; it's a natural occurrence. If an acorn falls on your head, would it hurt? Sure, a little, but a bump on the head doesn't constitute a crisis.

In the last chapter I explained comfort-food eating. Comfort food is that snuggly, cuddly, feel-good food. Stress food isn't about snugly, cuddly, feel-good food. It's about make-the-bad-feelings-go-away food. Stress food is eaten as self-medication. It's no different, really, from alcohol or drugs. At some point, you eat not to produce a specific good feeling but to make bad feelings go away. You'll gladly exchange a type of numbness for the stress you're feeling or the crisis you fear. Comfort eating brings in the good; stress eating blocks out the bad.

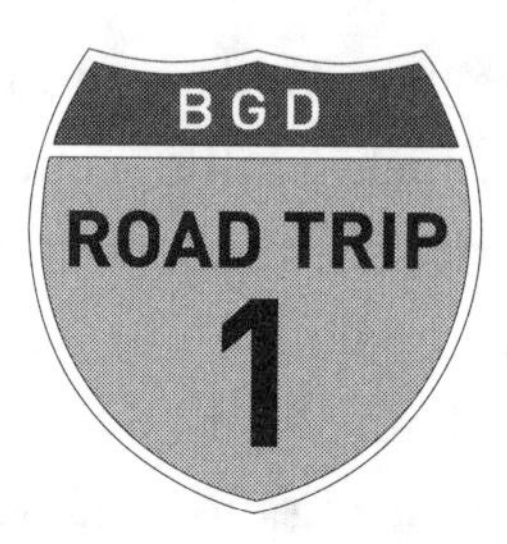

It's time for another inner journey. I want you to think about and write down the stressors you have in your life. These are your ongoing issues. Slam-on-the-brakes kind of things apply if they happen on a regular basis. You may be in a job where you're exposed to real emergencies. Even though this is "business as usual" for you, it's still stressful, so include your job on your list.

For the rest of you, your lists are probably going to include some chronic situations that arise from your families, your jobs, your health, your relationships, your finances, and your living situations. Here are some examples of what could be causing stress in your life:

- You're having an ongoing battle with a member of your family—a child, a parent, a spouse. Because they're family, you can't just get up and walk away, but being around this person is a real struggle.
- Work is just the pits. You need the job, but the conditions are intolerable. It's all you can do just to force yourself to go in each day. You keep hoping it's going to get better, but it never does.
- You have an ongoing health concern. Your doctor knows about it and is trying to treat it, but it doesn't seem to go away. It's a barrier to everything you want to do.
- There's never enough money. You're exhausted with trying to make ends meet. Every phone call, every letter in the mail could be somebody else haranguing you to pay up. You'd like to get away from it all, but getting away costs money, so there's nowhere to go.
- You're in the midst of a crisis of belief. God seems so distant. "Faith" is a foreign language you can barely make out. You keep waiting to feel better

spiritually so you can feel good about going back to church, but Sunday after Sunday goes by, and you just don't go.

- The past is a very real part of your present. An event or a situation in your past has a stranglehold on your present. You can't seem to get it out of your head and move on. Without closure, it festers as an open wound in your life.

Whatever is causing you stress, write it down on a list on the left-hand side of your paper.

God made stress a part of your life, but He does not want you to lead a stressful life. On the contrary, His plan for you is a life of joy and peace. You've panicked in your stress like the children of Israel and have been relying on your equivalent of a chocolate calf instead of God. The good news is there's nothing on your list that is impossible for God to handle. ♡

Succ-stress-ful Strategies

If stress is a fact of life, then you must come up with strategies for managing your stress that are meaningful for the long-term and that will draw you closer to God. When the people of Israel were stressed out about Moses on top of the mountain, they chose to react in rebellion and craft their own remedy. When you turn to stress eating, you are doing the same thing—choosing to react in rebellion to health and crafting your own remedy. Therefore, managing stress, and your weight by extension, becomes a spiritual issue. And unlike Chicken Little, you're *not* going to get ambushed by a sly fox along the way to the king! As you go over the following strategies for coping with stress, I want you to note (to the right of each appropriate stressor) any that relate to the specific stress situations you just wrote down during Road Trip #1.

Avoid stress triggers

Managing your stress is often a strategy of avoiding situations that are personally stressful. I, for example, would never take a part-time job at a Krispy Kreme store. If you can identify specific areas, situations, places, or people that cause you stress at this time in your life, you can minimize your exposure. For example, if your Uncle Roy drives you crazy arguing with Cousin Sally, don't invite them over to your house at the same time. If your mother always criticizes your housekeeping and never leaves a stone unturned when she comes to your house, why not arrange to meet her at a mall or a restaurant? If you don't have the money to go out to a movie and dinner with your friends, why not pack a picnic lunch and meet at the park for a meal and a nice long walk? If you know that a certain activity is a problem for you, steer clear until you are strong enough to face it. Here's advice from Proverbs 4:15 that can be applied to the stress from these situations: "Avoid it, do not pass by it; turn away from it and pass on" (NASU).

Redefine your stress

Falling acorns do not mean that the sky is falling. Look through your list of stressors. Can any of them be reevaluated? Is the fact that you're stressed out over being overweight really going to help you lose weight? Achieving the body God designed for you should be a source of excitement, anticipation, and motivation in your life, not a source of stress! You may not always be able to control your initial reaction, but you can choose your intentional response. Think of the times the people of Israel got it right when they entered the field of battle choosing to trust in God. Even though these were times of battle and a certain level of mayhem, they were counseled not to stress about it. If the people of Israel could enter that kind of battle without getting stressed out, so can we in our kind of battles.

Here are a couple of verses of encouragement from Deuteronomy 20:2–4: "When you are about to go into battle, the priest shall come forward and address the army. He shall say: 'Hear, O Israel, today you are going into battle against your enemies. Do not be fainthearted or afraid; do not be terrified or give way to panic before them. For the LORD your God is the one who goes with you to fight for you against your enemies to give you victory.'"

Lower your expectations

In the people I counsel, one of the greatest contributors to stress is their own expectations. They manufacture crises because life fails to meet their unrealistic expectations. This is a classic recipe for failure. If you lower your expectations to the range of the reachable, you will experience far less disappointment and frustration. Do you demand perfection? From yourself? Your spouse? Your children? Your family? Your job? Your health? This life doesn't come with guarantees, except one: it's not perfect. So stop wasting your time trying to achieve what is literally impossible. Your straining and stretching and trying and striving are producing a great deal of stress in your life. Aim instead for excellence in those rare moments when it's possible and for integrity when it's not. Remember that God's definition of great things is often doing the small things consistently and well.

Here's some instruction from Paul in Romans 12:3 that can help you adjust your expectations about yourself: "For through the grace given to me I say to everyone among you not to think more highly of himself than he ought to think; but to think so as to have sound judgment, as God has allotted to each a measure of faith" (NASU).

Think happy thoughts

It appears that the Julie Andrews character, Maria, in *The Sound of Music* was right; it does help to think of raindrops on roses and whiskers on kittens. This is also called *visualization*. It is an intentional strategy of choosing what you're going to mentally dwell on. If you always focus on the negative things in life, life will appear very negative, and this negative image is bound to cause you stress. After all, if you develop a "bunker" mentality to life, you will go around feeling under siege by the world. Since God is sovereign and Christ has conquered this world, you have a lot to be happy about.

Instead of focusing on the negative, intentionally choose to acknowledge the positive. Paul puts it pretty succinctly in Philippians 4:8: "Finally, brothers, whatever is true, whatever is noble, whatever is right, whatever is pure, whatever is lovely, whatever is admirable—if anything is excellent or praiseworthy—think about such things."

Banish worry

As a child, because you could intuit that your parents and other adults spent a lot of time worrying, you probably got the idea that "important people worry." You became an adult, and in the important role of "captain of your own destiny," you took on the attitudes and actions of other adults and began to worry. If you're a Christian, you might feel like you have even more to worry about than non-Christians because you are aware of the bigger picture, the unseen spiritual consequences connected to everyday experiences and world events.

And yet Jesus very specifically tells all of His followers not to worry. He doesn't want you to miss out on the most important component of that larger spiritual picture—the mighty power of God. Your struggle with your health and your weight has probably caused you to worry. God says you're to turn that worry over to Him.

Listen to Jesus in Matthew 6:25: "Therefore I tell you, do not worry about your life, what you will eat or drink; or about your body, what you will wear. Is not life more important than food, and the body more important than clothes?"

Take a walk

I've already talked about the benefits of physical activity and exercise. It just makes you feel better. When you are under stress, your body is poised for either fight or flight. In order to help it adjust back to normal, do something physical. Talk a walk, ride your bike, mow the yard, clean the house, play ball with your kids, or take the dog for a walk. If you're under a pretty big load of stress on an ongoing basis, it will be important for you to engage daily in moderate, physical exercise to help manage that stress. Not only will you work off some of that adrenaline, but you'll also be helping yourself get better sleep because of the natural fatigue that happens with physical activity. Since stress can cause you to isolate yourself from others, physical activity allows you to get out and engage in the world around you. Thank God for the beauty He's made and allowed you to participate in.

Here are your marching orders from Genesis 13:17: "Go, walk through the length and breadth of the land, for I am giving it to you."

Have a talk

It's good to be able to talk things over with trusted and trustworthy friends. Now, by talking, I don't mean venting or raging or railing against life. I mean talking things out with a wise friend or family member. You'll need to use some discernment in choosing the right person. I know people I could go to with a small problem who would have me convinced by the end of our time that all was lost and there was no hope left in the world. Choose positive, encouraging people to talk with, those who are spiritually mature and can help guide you to greater understanding of God's Word, hope, and love in the world.

Ideally, you want those who can relate to your situation and to your stress and who can help model how they overcame or are coping with a similar situation. If you don't really have a family member or friend you can go to, consider working with a Christian therapist. (No, this is not a shameless plug for my business. It is, however, a shameless plug for my line of work, which I very much believe in, and I know of changed lives to prove it!) You need others to guide, encourage, and hold you accountable.

Here's a reminder from Ecclesiastes 4:12: "Though one may be overpowered, two can defend themselves. A cord of three strands is not quickly broken."

Journal

No, I'm not going to tell you to start a "Dear Diary." However, journaling is what you've been doing throughout this book. Journaling is writing down your thoughts and plans. It's a way to see your mind in print. This might appear to be a daunting prospect, but journals can be kept strictly confidential, so don't worry! If you're faced with a difficult, unavoidable situation, one way to relieve stress is to express your feelings about it on paper for only yourself to see. A good practice, if you are really angry about something and having a hard time letting go of that anger, is to write down your negative feelings and thoughts on a piece of paper. Then, destroy the piece of paper and allow yourself to release those thoughts with it.

Now, before some of you start saying, "Oh, come on! How can that be effective?" just trust me on this. Some of the stress you carry around is from people and situations that are in the past and cannot be "fixed." They are what they are and you must move forward. Writing down what you weren't able to say at the time and have no opportunity to say now, then releasing those thoughts, can be a very freeing experience, especially if done in conjunction with prayer.

You can even journal your thoughts about God to God. And don't worry; there is ample precedence in Scripture for this very thing. It's called the Book of Psalms, and David was pretty up front with God in many of the psalms he wrote. God not only accepted David's thoughts, but He also caused them to be included in His Bible. God, our King, is big enough to accept your thoughts, too.

Listen to how honest David was with God in Psalm 43:1–2: "Declare me innocent, O God! Defend me against these ungodly people. Rescue me from these unjust liars. For you are God, my only safe haven. Why have you tossed me aside? Why must I wander around in grief, oppressed by my enemies?" (NLT).

The words of David's son, Solomon, in Proverbs 16:13 also remind you that your King wants you to be honest with Him: "Kings take pleasure in honest lips; they value a man who speaks the truth."

Tell yourself to relax

As weird as it sounds, sometimes you have to tell yourself to relax. You need to remind yourself to knock it off when you're getting tense and stressed. Breathing deeply and regularly can help us relax since often we can hyperventilate when under stress, causing that light-headed, disconnected feeling (to say nothing of passing out altogether).

Stretching your muscles and rotating your head, neck, and shoulders can help reduce physical stress. If Chicken Little had told herself, "Relax; it's just an acorn!" then Chicken Little, Henny Penny, Ducky Lucky, Goosey Loosey, and Turkey Lurkey would not have fallen for Foxy Loxy. In fact, that might be a good thing for you to say to yourself: "Relax; it's just an acorn." You need to ask God to help you see that fallen acorn for what it truly is.

Here is a promise from James 1:5 that God will give you that kind of wisdom: "If any of you lacks wisdom, he should ask God, who gives generously to all without finding fault, and it will be given to him."

Be creative

Hopefully you've already come up with some creative ways to deal with your own stress, and that's one aspect of what I mean by this heading. The other aspect is for you to *be* creative—paint, play an instrument, sing, sculpt, write (I've talked about journaling, but now I'm talking about poetry or prose), listen to music, even garden. These are all activities that allow you to experience the joy of your aesthetic side.

In our treatment models at the Center, we have specific times set aside for people to sing, to draw, to listen to music, and to make small art projects. These activities allow us to use other areas of our brains to tap into our creative selves. They are very powerful and can help us find our way back to joy. When we are involved in creative activities, we're engaged in life. Then stress has a harder time finding a foothold.

I can think of few things more stressful than what Paul and Silas experienced. They'd gone to the city of Philippi and found themselves afoul of the owners of a slave girl who kept following them around for days yelling after them. Finally, Paul had had enough, and he banished the evil spirit from the girl. This was good for her, but bad for her owners. This spirit had enabled the girl to tell the future, and the girl's owners were making money from this poor child's possessed state. The owners, deprived of their livelihood, initiated a riot. Paul and his companion Silas were attacked, stripped, severely flogged, and thrown into prison. All in all, it must have been a pretty stressful couple of days.

But here's how Paul and Silas dealt with their stress in a very creative and surprising way, one that all of us can emulate: "About midnight Paul and Silas were praying and singing hymns to God, and the other prisoners were listening to them" (Acts 16:25).

Pray and be still

Now we will discuss the last strategy—last but certainly not least. Pray and be still. In fact, all of the strategies above are made more effective if prayer is a part. When God is a reality in your life, His presence and promises form a hedge of protection around you. When stress threatens to overwhelm, prayer can bring you back into focus. This chapter started out with a simple verse: "Be still, and know that I am God." It really all comes back to that, where so many things in life are concerned, including and perhaps especially where stress is concerned.

The opposite of stress is peace. When you rest in the Lord and are confident in who He is in your life, you can have peace, even in the midst of stress. At midnight, after a horrific day, Paul and Silas were able to have peace.

It is from that city where they were beaten and jailed that Paul writes the following words about the power of prayer to bring peace to our lives: "Do not be anxious about anything, but in everything, by prayer and petition, with thanksgiving, present your requests to God. And the peace of God, which transcends all understanding, will guard your hearts and your minds in Christ Jesus" (Philippians 4:6–7).

Did you catch what that verse said? You're not to be anxious about *anything*. I have to be honest here and say that I'm not there yet. There are things in my life I do get anxious about, and those things cause stress in my life. The goal here is not be able to stand up like a superhero (you know the stance—legs slightly apart, chest out, chin up, hands on your hips, a determined look in your eyes) and declare myself perfect when it comes to anxiety and stress. I'm a person, not a spiritual superhero; I'm a spiritual work in progress. My goal is to keep working toward turning over my anxieties to God in order to allow His peace to establish small beachheads on the shores of stress. (OK, it may seem a little strange to use battle language when talking about peace, but this really is a battle for me, and for you, too, if you're honest. I'm just being honest for all of us.)

The Saga of the Seeds

Yes, it's a battle, and there are forces arrayed against you that do not want you to win the battle over stress. Stress may be physical and psychological in this life, but it has long-reaching complications in the next. Stress and worry can rob you of your joy and your ability to absorb and grow in God's Word. In case you think this is a recent phenomenon, given our hectic, crazy, frenetic pace of twenty-first-century life, think again. Jesus addressed this issue over two thousand years ago in an interesting parable about seeds.

In Luke 8, Jesus tells the story of a farmer who goes out to sow seeds in his fields. Some of the seed fell along the pathway next to the field. That seed got trampled and eaten up by birds because it was exposed. As the farmer continued to throw out the seed, part of it wound up in rocky soil where it germinated, but the young plants ended up withering and dying in the heat because they didn't have a good root system established in the rocky soil. Still more seed fell into thorny soil where it also germinated, but the young plants couldn't compete with the more aggressive weeds. Of course, the seed that landed on the *good* soil germinated and produced a lush crop. ("Oh, how quaint," you say. "An agricultural tale. But how does that have any relevance in our current situation? After all, I'm not a farmer!")

Remember, the story is a parable; it has a very relevant application. And don't feel bad if you had trouble finding the relevance; the disciples who heard it didn't understand it either and needed Jesus to explain:

> This is the meaning of the parable: The seed is the word of God. Those along the path are the ones who hear, and then the devil comes and takes away the word from their hearts, so that they may not believe and be saved. Those on the rock are the ones who receive the word with joy when they hear it, but they have no root. They believe for a while, but in the time of testing they fall away. The seed that fell among thorns stands for those who hear, but as they go on their way they are choked by life's worries, riches and pleasures, and they do not mature. But the seed on good soil stands for those with a noble and good heart, who hear the word, retain it, and by persevering produce a crop.
>
> —Luke 8:11–15

Yes, you heard it right. When you allow stress a foothold in your life, you teeter dangerously close to becoming the third type of seed—the kind that is choked by life's worries, riches, and pleasure, those who don't mature in Christ. Yes, putting on pounds because of stress is a reality, but the real damage of stress is a lack of maturity in Christ.

You must ask God to weed your soil and help you remove the thorns of worry and care that choke out His Word so that it cannot affect your life. When you do this, your soil will improve, and you'll begin to produce as God intended. By overcoming the effects of stress, you can have victory over your stress eating, which keeps you in that thorny soil and which keeps you from achieving the body God designed for you.

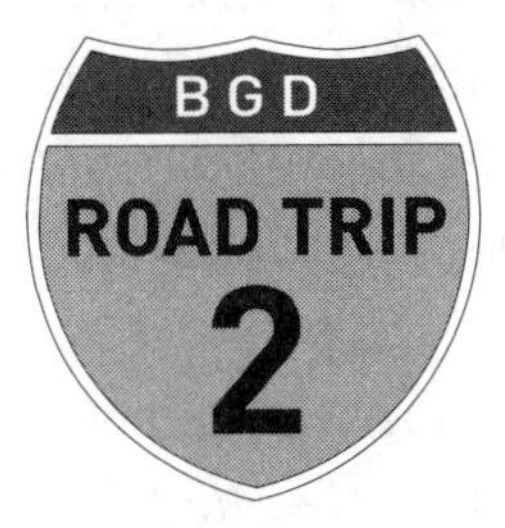

Now that you have your list of what causes stress in your life, I want you to pray through the list. I want you to go down each stress, confess it to God, and ask for His help in overcoming that stress. There are a myriad of reasons to do this, including the toll stress and stress eating take on the body God designed for you. You were meant to experience the amazing peace of God through Christ. When you surrender to stress, you declare to the world that God is not big enough to handle your worries and your strife. You know in your mind this isn't true, but you must feel it in your heart so you can live it in your life as a witness to God's power and provision. God has promised to guard both hearts and minds in Christ.

After you've prayed through your list, I have an optional activity for you. Take a walk. Paint a picture. Write a poem. Go rent a copy of *The Sound of Music* and sing along. Get out and enjoy life—that's the best stress reliever of all and a gift of God.

Oh, for a life free from stress! Lord, I confess I've allowed worry and the cares of this life to strangle my joy and witness for You. Guard my heart and my mind in Christ, and give me peace in my life. I so long for peace. I confess I have not trusted You to give it to me. Instead, I have reached for things to put in my mouth, trying to hold the stress at bay. I also confess that it did not work. I'm still stressed and carrying more weight than You designed for my body. I commit today, Father, to purposefully give over my stresses to You. I commit to turning to You in prayer and engaging in uplifting, positive activities to relieve my stress instead of turning to food. Fill me with joy in Your presence, Lord. Fill me up so I need nothing more! Amen.

Chapter 10

I'll Take the Crown but Not the Gray

> Gray hair is a crown of splendor; it is attained by a righteous life.
>
> —Proverbs 16:31

No discussion of health and weight would be complete without talking about what happens as we age. For many of us, hitting forty is like hitting a wall going forty miles per hour. Overnight our bodies appear to deteriorate before our very eyes. If gray hair is a crown, then stretch marks, liver spots, and wrinkles are the crown jewels most of us would rather do without!

I am uniquely qualified to talk about this subject because I have gray hair. Actually, I've had gray hair since my early thirties. It's just a part of who I am, and I don't really think about it much. I don't think other people really give it much thought either, although it may have seemed odd fifteen years ago. Now, if all of a sudden I showed up at work after a vacation with jet-black hair, *that* would be strange! I could probably become the perfect poster child for Grecian Formula because of my age demographic, but I've never considered covering up my gray hair. At my age now, in my late forties, I'm a bit of an anomaly, if the shelves at the grocery store are any indication. There are rows and rows, boxes and boxes, of all types of hair-coloring products for men and for women. Somewhere along the line, gray hair has become a source of embarrassment instead of "a crown of splendor."

Gray hair, for most people, is a sign of aging. Since this is anathema to our culture, we cover it up. We have creams for our liver spots, dermal abrasion for our stretch marks, and Botox for our wrinkles. We work very hard to obscure the fact that we're aging. One of the most stubborn side effects of aging is the weight gain that happens as we age.

Middle-Age Spread

Our bodies, as we age, go into a sort of reverse puberty. Remember puberty? Most of us have spent years trying to forget it, but take a time-out and think back to your early adolescence. As you transitioned from child to young adult, you underwent some pretty amazing changes, both physical and emotional. This was probably a time of fervent prayer in your household—by your parents!

Adolescents are challenging. Just ask any middle-school or high-school teacher. As their bodies are adjusting, one day can be literally night-and-day different from the next. The people around teens tend to give them plenty of space. When someone asks their parents how old their kids are and they answer thirteen or fourteen or fifteen, there are plenty of nodding heads and knowing looks, along with comments like, "Don't worry; it won't last forever, even though it *seems* like it will," or "Wow! Know what you mean!" or "My kids are grown, thank God!"

Universally, we seem to understand that adolescence is a time of change and that adolescents need to be given a certain amount of slack. No such grace is given when it comes to the flip side of puberty—the physical and emotional changes that occur as we transition from adulthood to older adulthood. After all, we're adults, so we're supposed to enter this time in our lives stoically. Just shut up and don't complain.

Well, as uninformed as many adolescents are about puberty, I find a similar lack of understanding about the aging process, especially about the middle-aging process. Perhaps it's because I'm right there myself, but I also think it goes back up to the whole gray-hair/hair-dye thing. We don't talk about aging because we're trying so very, very hard to pretend it doesn't exist!

But I'm going to talk about it now because it has relevance to our discussion of the body God designed for you. His perfect design isn't "one age fits all." Aging is a part of His plan for your body.

Let's take a look at some of the changes that occur as we age. In keeping with the Bible verse at the beginning of this chapter, I'll start at the head and move down from there. (I said "down," not "downhill." Let's at least try to keep a positive attitude through this, shall we?)

- Our hair begins to turn gray and thin. Sometimes, it thins out into nothingness, also called hair loss.
- Our brains don't produce as many neurons as when we were young. We have more trouble remembering. (I'm in real trouble where my keys are concerned!)
- Our eyes produce less tears. Our eyes don't focus as well as they used to. It can become difficult to see clearly up close as the retinas thin and our lenses cloud.
- Our ears are more sensitive to damage and hearing loss. We tend to say "What?" and "Pardon me?" more often.

- Our mouths can be drier. We can become "long in the tooth," as our gums recede. The accumulated wear and tear on our teeth can cause chips and breaks.
- Our skin develops age spots and is generally drier and less elastic. We develop wrinkles.
- Our bones become more brittle and fracture more easily.
- The heart muscle can begin to work less efficiently. Depending upon our heredity and dietary habits, our arteries can develop fatty deposits that compromise our hearts and circulatory system and lead to high blood pressure.
- Our digestive system becomes more sluggish and can result in increased constipation.
- Our kidneys may not work as well, and the muscles holding in our urine can weaken, causing urinary incontinence.
- Our waistlines expand—enough said for now.
- Our libido shifts more into neutral.
- A good night's sleep can be harder to come by. We sleep less and less well.

There, that wasn't so bad, was it?

OK, it's easy to see why people don't want to think about aging. Taken to the extreme, this is hardly a pretty picture. Now, while aging is inevitable, there is a great deal you can do to mitigate and gracefully ride the wave of these effects instead of being dragged down in the undertow of decline.

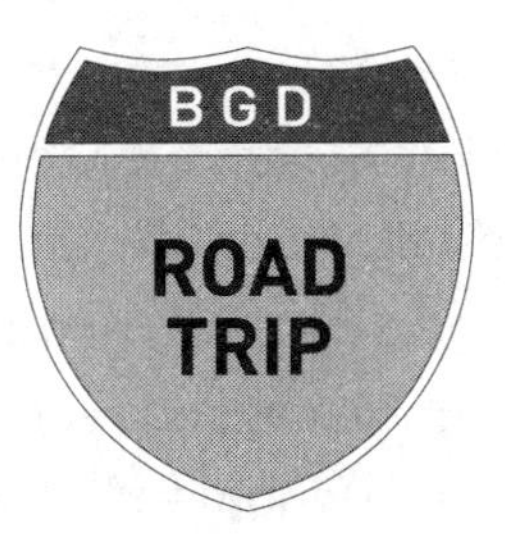

Before you read any further, I want you to go to the bathroom. Not to actually go to the bathroom, unless you need to, of course, which is fine. But I want you to go to the bathroom because that's where most people have a large mirror. Do you remember the courage it took at the start of this book to really look at yourself in the mirror? Well, I want you to hoist up your courage again and go back to that mirror. This time, I want you to look in the mirror and examine the ways you're aging. Look at yourself from all angles. In what way does your body reveal your current age? How has your body changed in the last ten years? Five years? In the last year?

Now, please answer this question:

How do you feel about your body right now?

Honestly, you might be pretty frustrated or mad or disappointed with your body. You may want to look at your body as the enemy. This thinking must STOP! Your body is not your enemy. It's not your body's fault that you're aging. Every new gray hair, wrinkle, or liver spot is not a cause for panic. Aging is not the sky falling; aging is an acorn dropping—it is a natural occurrence. It is not a crisis.

When you take a natural, God-designed function and make it a crisis, you send a message to everyone around you that you don't really trust in God. When you allow age to devalue you as an individual, you join in with the foolish thinking of society rather than the wisdom of God's Word. When you give in to despair and hopelessness because of your aging, you surrender to the true enemy. Wrinkles are not your enemy; the deceiver is. (In case you don't know whom I'm talking about, Satan is the deceiver. The Bible calls him the father of lies, and he is the one who fuels the lies about value and worth being wrapped up in a youthful package.)

After you've written down all of your personal aging effects, I also want you to write a letter of acceptance of your age and your trust in God for today and tomorrow. It could be something like this:

> I, [your name here], accept my age. I thank You, God, for the gift of life today to be this age. I trust You to take care of me today. I ask You to allow me to age into tomorrow.

Body Serenity

This is a perfect time to remember the Body Serenity Prayer from the introduction of this book. (You didn't just skim the introduction, did you, thinking that since it was the "introduction" it wouldn't contain anything really valuable? For those of you who did read it through, congratulations and my thanks!) The Body Serenity Prayer was my adaptation of the original Serenity Prayer, and it goes like this:

God, grant me the serenity to accept the things about my body I cannot change, the courage to change the things I can for the better, and the wisdom to know the difference and get on with my life. Amen.

This prayer and these sentiments are going to be relevant for you as you age. There will be aspects about aging you cannot change; they are God designed. No amount of cosmetic, bariatric, or other surgery is going to change them. You've already encountered the courage it takes to make positive changes in your life. With prayer, patience, and practice, you're gaining the wisdom from God to know the difference. Let's go back to the rather distressing list of aging effects and see how you can put the Body Serenity Prayer into practice.

Crowned with splendor

How and when your hair grays or falls out is determined by genetics. Your genetics are part of your original equipment (again, from the introduction; see how important it was for you to read it?). Granted, hair can fall out because of an illness or medical treatment, but that's not what I'm addressing here. I'm talking about the normal thinning of your hair that happens as you age.

What can you do about gray or thinning hair?

I'm really not opposed to people coloring their hair, regardless of what I said at the beginning of this chapter. If you think red or brown or green hair reflects who you are, then go for it! My concern is with those who choose to run away from their gray hair out of a sense of dread or denial. Coloring your hair because you want it to be a certain color is much better than coloring it just to cover up the gray because you're embarrassed by it. Aging is nothing to be embarrassed about; that's the world talking, and you need to tell it to quiet down.

For some people, natural gray hair may be much more attractive than artificially colored hair. Several years ago, a wonderful lady attended the same church I did. She had jet-black hair the entire time I had known her, and now she was well into her sixties. It was obvious she colored her hair. People of her ethnic background do not have jet-black hair in their sixties. Unfortunately, she developed cancer, and she lost her hair during the chemotherapy. When it came back in, her hair was the most beautiful gray I've ever seen. Before, all I noticed was that shock of black hair; now I could see this regal face literally crowned in silver. Before she got sick, she used to wear it in a (how do I say this?) 1950s' flip style. After the chemotherapy, she wore her hair in an attractive shorter cut that complimented her face. Rather than being a negative, her hair had become a positive. Now she was free from the nagging concern over those blasted gray roots that constantly peeked out at the top of her head. Her granddaughters chided her for hiding her beautiful hair all that time!

It's worth noting that sometimes your hair thins because you're not getting the nutrients you need. By eating well and taking your multivitamin and other supplements, you can help your body have the building blocks it needs to continue to produce healthy hair as long as your genes are designed to do it. There's no reason to quicken the pace!

I recognize there are those who undergo noninvasive techniques or even surgical procedures to enhance the amount of hair they have. Some of these can be draconian. I know of a man who had the top of his skull sliced in two so that bald skin could be removed. This caused the two sides of his head, which had hair, to come closer together (you can see where he was going with this). When I heard about it, my first thought was, "What were you thinking?" The second was that this must have been extraordinarily painful, which he readily conceded, saying that had he known how painful it was going to be, he never would have done it in the first place. Vanity is one thing; pain is something completely different. I'll allow that to stand as a warning to whoever chooses to listen. The third thing I thought about was the scar. What happens if he continues to lose his hair, even the parts on the sides he has now? Won't there be a tremendous scar running lengthwise down the top of his head? That would constitute a problem. How would you cover up something like that?

Finding your keys, part 2

I've already told you I have trouble remembering where I put things. This forgetfulness, which begins initially because of too many things on my mind, can turn into not enough things in my mind as the number of neurons my brain produces decreases. This forgetfulness in aging is jokingly referred to as having a "senior moment." I don't remember hearing this phrase when I was younger. But as soon as I started heading toward fifty, whenever I forgot anything, I started hearing, "Ah, a senior moment." These were almost always spoken by an older person, who smiled warmly at me in solidarity. Frankly, I wasn't pleased with that observation at first. "What? I'm not a senior citizen! Why, that's like saying I look 'fatter in flesh'!" Then upon calm reflection, I thought, "OK, good; if they recognize this as a sign of aging, then it's not just me!"

Now, I don't plan to coast into neural never-never land without a fight. Again, it's important to maintain a healthy diet and supplementation. Your brain is organic and needs fuel to operate. Go back to the fat chapter and reread all the potential benefits to taking essential fatty acids. Several of them had to do with increased cognitive function. If you're not taking a fish oil supplement, think again (and your keys will thank you).

There's another important aspect to this forgetfulness phenomenon, and it was discussed in the last chapter. When you are stressed out and operating at maximum capacity mentally, physically, and emotionally, your tendency to forget things will naturally increase.

The first things to suffer under chronic stress are your ability to remember things and to maintain emotional equilibrium. By dialing down my stress factor (and not trying to concentrate on five disparate things as I'm getting ready for work), I might actually have a calm moment to remember back to where I did put my keys the night before. Stress puts me on autopilot, which means I'm not taking the time to notice my world in the here and now. When I do that, my keys are history, and I have to call LaFon to borrow her set so I can get to work.

Another strategy I have employed is writing things down. I used to be able to keep my schedule swirling around like a swarm of events right above my head. Anytime I needed to remember something, I'd just mentally reach up and pull down the pertinent fact. It was always there at my fingertips, swirling about my head, ready to be used. Well, the swarm has flown the coop. Now I know and accept that I need to write down what I'm doing and when. I don't fight against this, but I accept it gladly with the help of technology.

I'm a bit of a gadget guy. I love technology and little electronic devices. I'm so grateful to God that I was born in this age of PDAs and computers because I just love the darn things. (Luckily, I was also born as the son of my father, Larry, who doesn't just love all this technological stuff, he also *understands* it. He handles all of our technology resources at the Center, and there isn't a day that goes by that I'm not grateful he's my dad! I'm also the father of a seven-year-old techno-wonder, who already appears to have a neuroconnection with all things computer. I'm sandwiched between electronic wizards!)

Instead of bemoaning the fact that you can't remember dates and events, create a system to help you remember. Sure, it could be something as Neanderthal as a pocket calendar. Or it could be something high tech and amazing! Once you accept the fact that you need the help, there are many ways to tailor a solution that not only takes care of the issue but also reflects your tastes and personality. Then it's *you* taking control over your schedule instead of vice versa.

Cry me a river

A couple of years ago, I started seeing a commercial on television for a product that helps your body produce more tears. Dry eyes can also be an effect of aging, along with the loss of ability to focus your vision. All of a sudden, people who have never worn glasses in their lives have trouble reading newsprint six inches away. Now you know why bifocals were invented and why pharmacies sell racks of them. As you age, your eyes become less flexible, and your ability to adjust from near to far or far to near is compromised.

It's odd, but I've found that people's eyes are a source of denial when it comes to aging. First, they doggedly put off getting reading glasses if they've never worn glasses before. And if they have worn glasses before, they resist the suggestion that they need bifocals or trifocals. Why? Because these products are associated with aging. So, they fight against them. Frankly, I like my glasses. I don't use them much, but when I do, they're very helpful.

If your eyes are dry, use eye drops. Having trouble reading? Get glasses. These are perfectly legitimate, logical fixes. Again, these are not crises; they're addressable issues. It is not reasonable to expect the normal, physiological changes of aging to miraculously pass you by. You could be running a marathon every other weekend and be in better shape than a twenty-year-old marine and still need reading glasses or eye drops at forty-five. I think you'll find that once you've provided yourself with a solution, you'll stop focusing on the problem.

Say what?

As you age, your ears become less forgiving. The accumulated damage of all those Grateful Dead concerts and stereos turned up loud comes home to roost. An aging rocker talks about his near deafness now because of the high decibels he experienced during his career. His message to a generation of musicians and music lovers is to treat our ears more kindly—and turn that music down!

At this point in life, I'm surprised at how loud my world has become. With two small boys at home, with radio, television, electronic games all blaring, it can be overwhelming. I'm reminded of the need for quiet time before God in the midst of the din. I think, though, that we need silence for other times in our lives, too. Just turning down the noise level of our lives can lead to reduced stress as well.

But as I age, if there comes a time when it is difficult to understand what is happening around me, I'll get a hearing aid, and I'll give thanks to God for the amazing technology that allows me to hear clearly again. For so many of these effects of aging, we live in a blessed time, when science and technology are providing viable solutions. Instead of begrudging your need for a hearing aid, give thanks to God that you're able to even have such a thing available. How you handle the effects of aging has a lot to do with your attitude. Gracefully aging or aging *with grace* has meaning on several levels.

Open wide

When is the last time you went to the dentist? Are you experiencing dry mouth or receding gums or chipped teeth or tooth pain? Go to the dentist! These conditions are not going to go away on their own. Some will only become progressively worse.

I have a great dentist. He's both a dentist and a friend. We have worked together to restore the teeth of eating disorder patients, and I can't say enough about his professionalism, care, and expertise. I understand some people have a real fear of dentists. The staff members at my dentist's office go out of their way to help assuage those fears and help their patients be comfortable and at ease with dental procedures. There are dentists out there who understand your fears and will be as accommodating as they possibly can be. I promise.

Go to the dentist and save your teeth. (For those of you so inclined, go and get your teeth whitened. It isn't something that lasts forever, but it can certainly give you a boost.) Whatever the state of your mouth, your dentist can help suggest strategies to minimize future damage and correct past problems. Even though your teeth are original equipment, there is much that can be done today to protect this valuable asset.

Skin deep

Did you know that your skin is classified as an organ? It's pretty amazing, really. Think of all the wear and tear and exposure it endures over the years. Some of us are harder on our skin than others. When I was growing up in Idaho, sunbathing was popular, especially in the summer. It was considered healthy to have a tan. Nowadays, we know the dangers of sun exposure, and sunscreen is a prerequisite for any Jantz family summer outing.

As you age, your skin can become drier and less elastic. It doesn't "spring" back as easily or handle harsh elements as forgivingly. You get wrinkles. It's a mantra, but I'll say it again—eat a healthy diet and take your supplements. As an organ, your skin is looking to you to provide it with the nutrients it needs to repair itself and stay vibrant.

Protect your skin with lotions and sunscreen. If the age spots bother you, use a moisturizing makeup. All of this, of course, should be done within moderation and proper perspective. If the goal is to impress, it will be of limited value. Scripture is quite specific that these activities done for vain purposes profit you nothing. Your goal should be to enhance the health and vitality of your skin, not to try to look like someone you're not. Enhance what you have; don't hide who you are.

Sticks and stones

Bone density is very important. It's determined by genetics, but it can be affected by environmental factors and some medications. The loss of bone density can bring about a condition known as osteoporosis. Whether you are a man or a woman, osteoporosis is a reality that must be addressed as you age. There are ways to combat osteoporosis that everyone can do regardless of age. Make sure you're getting the appropriate amount of calcium for your age, condition, and gender. This is something you can coordinate with your physician. You can even take a bone density test to see what the condition of your bones is right now. Without testing, osteoporosis isn't something people are aware of ahead of time. Rather, it slowly creeps up on a person, so it's good to be forewarned, and bone density testing can help.

Besides getting the right amount of calcium, make sure you exercise. Weight-bearing exercise helps keep your bones strong and healthy. It's just one more great reason to get out and become active! This is especially true for women who are menopausal. The lowering of your estrogen levels can negatively impact the rate at which your body naturally loses bone density because of aging. If you are at a higher risk for osteoporosis (women more than men; small-boned women more than larger-boned women; Asian or Caucasian more than African American), make sure this is something you're watching with your doctor.

The beat goes on

Your heart beats an average of 70 beats a minute every day of your life. If you're forty years old, it's already beaten 1,471,680,000 times. Every year, it adds almost 37 million beats to that total—all without you having to do anything. The beating of your heart is autonomic; it's an involuntary movement. It's also an elegant design of God. Your heart is at the heart, if you will, of your original equipment.

You, as an end user, however, are able to make modifications to your heart. The biggest modification you can make is through the foods you eat. I've already talked about the bad fats, those producing fatty deposits that line and clog up your arteries. Symptoms related to these modifications can occur in middle age through heart attacks or heart conditions.

You're really doing your heart a favor by reducing excess weight. Your heart has to work harder to support that excess fat—extra blood vessels need to support it, and it takes extra energy to move it from place to place. Your heart has to work harder to move two hundred pounds from point A to point B than it would if you weighed one hundred fifty pounds. By eating well and reducing or eliminating trans fats and saturated fats, you're lowering your cholesterol levels and avoiding the fatty buildup in your arteries. When your heart is strong and healthy, it will power your body for many, many years. Of course, only God knows the number of your days, but you can help protect the quality of those days by being proactive now in how you care for your health and your heart.

Plugged up

It is a cliché of laxative ads to have an older couple harping on each other about being constipated. Usually, this nagging takes place with a loud voice in front of a crowd of people. As you age, your digestive system can work less effectively, causing constipation. And along with the discomfort of constipation comes cramping, gas, and bloating. Who wants to deal with that? But this doesn't necessarily need to be your fate if you're older. There are things you can do today to help things progress smoothly internally.

Remember your meal-tracking worksheet and how many vegetables and fruits are on it? (Yes, the meal-tracking worksheet—the one you're supposed to be using daily to track what you eat, remember?

Just because I haven't mentioned it in a while doesn't mean I've forgotten about it. You need to be writing down what you eat as part of your baby steps to achieving the body God designed for you!) One of the benefits of eating all those fruits and veggies is the dietary fiber they provide. This dietary fiber gives your digestive system something to work with and move through your bowels. Whole grains are also an excellent source of dietary fiber. You can also use a fiber supplement, but make sure it is one that is free from any sort of stimulant. Look for one that is made of the plant fiber psyllium. Fiber supplements are a natural way to make sure you have the bulk you need in your gut to keep the presses rolling!

It all depends

Incontinence is generally not a normal condition of middle age. However, as you age, the muscles that control your urinary functions can weaken and cause urinary incontinence. (If you're a younger person, you may have a different condition known as overactive bladder. That's different and can be helped through medication. A trip to your doctor can determine if it's aging or a medical condition.) Urinary incontinence is sometimes called stress incontinence, where the stress of a sneeze or cough will result in leakage. Because this is caused by muscle weakness, especially for women who have given birth vaginally, it can be improved with exercise. Now, I personally have no experience with Kegel exercises, but my wife, LaFon, does. These are the pelvic exercises a woman will usually be instructed to do during and after pregnancy to strengthen the muscles that hold in the bladder, uterus, and rectum, also called the pelvic floor. (For the scientifically curious, there's good information about the pelvic floor at "Your Body's Design for Bladder Control" [http://kidney.niddk.nih.gov/kudiseses/pubs/bodydesign_ez], a Web site brought to you by the National Institutes of Health—your tax dollars at work, this time for the sake of your bladder!)

I suggest you actively work with your primary care physician to address this issue if you are experiencing stress incontinence. There is a whole range of strategies you can use, from dietary changes to physical exercises, such as the Kegel exercises, to pharmaceutical responses. (You'll need to watch alcohol and caffeine consumption because alcohol relaxes muscles and is a mild diuretic, and caffeine is both a diuretic and a stimulant that gets your bladder working overtime.)

The vast wasteland (or was that waistband?)

You know you're getting older when the section where you shop at the department store has pants with elastic waistbands. Just think about that. Junior sections don't have pants with elastic waistbands. If you see elastic waistbands, you're either in the children's department or the older folks' department.

It doesn't matter if you're male or female. Well, I take that back; the approach varies a little. If you're a woman, they put the elastic in the back of the pants. If you're a man, they just factor in more inches in your waist and call it a "relaxed fit." There's nothing relaxing about trying on stiff blue jeans with a waist size too small! For men's dress slacks, they'll often put in a short piece of elastic right near the front fastener to allow the pants to "breathe" with you. However you want to slice it, abdominal fat is often a companion of middle age.

Before you beat yourself up about it, realize that some of this weight gain is preloaded into your design. For women, it centers around menopause. For men, it centers around andropause. *Andropause* means low testosterone and is also called male menopause. Let's talk about it for a minute. In an article in 2001, two researchers from the Institute of Endocrinology and Medicine in Atlanta, Georgia, reported that 40 percent of men they surveyed age forty and above reported the following symptoms:[1]

- Lethargy or fatigue
- Depression
- Increased irritability
- Mood swings
- Loss of bone density
- Decrease in lean muscle
- Increase in fat
- Anemia or low iron
- Decreased libido
- Difficulty with erections

I think that pretty much outlines "male menopause." These are real issues even if the medical community hasn't put a specific name on them until now. So women are not the only ones who deal with the hormonal and physiological changes of age. For women, it's the loss of estrogen and progesterone; for men, it's the loss of testosterone. Testosterone, progesterone, and estrogen are combined in differing amounts in both men and women. With younger women, estrogen is high. With younger men, testosterone is high. However, as we age, estrogen drops in women and testosterone drops in men. Older women can sometimes have a higher ratio of testosterone than their husbands. And older men can have a higher ratio of estrogen than their wives.

Let's talk about women and estrogen now. In menopause, when estrogen levels drop, the body attempts to compensate for this loss by producing abdominal fat. Abdominal fat is an alternative source of estrogen. It is, therefore, no surprise that middle-aged women need elastic waistbands, as their bodies are predisposed to put on this abdominal fat. Men, on the other hand, as they lose testosterone, increase their ratio of estrogen. Because testosterone is dropping, lean muscle production is reduced, so their metabolism slows down. (Lean muscle is a roaring furnace for metabolism, burning up fat and calories.) As their metabolism slows down, their conversion of excess calories to fat increases, and so does their waist size.

So, we're all in this together, both men and women, as we age. Because of that, each of us should be considerate and compassionate with each other.

Remember when I talked earlier about being a baby boomer? Boomers handle aging issues a little bit differently than generations past. In Seattle, a musical just closed that had been playing for almost two years. It was called *Menopause: The Musical.* One of my female colleagues went to see the show, and she loved it. (She just turned fifty this year.) She said she knew she was at the right place for the show when she drove up and saw a stream of middle-aged women converging on the Washington State Convention Center where the theater was located.

Apparently, *Menopause: The Musical* is a humorous look at the classic female symptoms of menopause (hot flashes, night sweats, irritability, memory lapses, lack of sleep—sounds like a fun show, doesn't it?). The plot of the show is four women who meet at a department store and forge a friendship around their menopausal symptoms. (At this point, I was nodding but not quite visualizing how this could be considered a comedy.) Taking songs from the '60s and '70s, each symptom was heralded, such as "Having a Hot Flash, a Tropical Hot Flash" or "Change of Life" (instead of "Chain of Fools").

After I got over my initial reaction, I thought how interesting it was that boomer women were confronting this physiological change with humor and acceptance. I'm fairly sure *Andropause: The Musical* is not in preproduction somewhere, but that doesn't mean men can't be alert to and aware of the changes our own bodies undergo as we age.

Whether you are male or female, one of the best ways to handle and navigate these changes is to be proactive about your body. One of the best things you can do is to reduce your excess fat. For women, this is vital because abdominal fat is not good fat; it's fat that sits around the major organs. (Remember the apple people in the first chapter?) The leaner a woman is, the less abdominal fat her organs have to contend with. For men, it's the same song, second verse. For male abdominal fat, think "beer belly" without the brew.

Exercise is an excellent way for you to maximize your lean muscle and help elevate your metabolism. This is true whatever your gender or age. So, stay active and keep yourself fit. This will help with your overall weight, and the exercise will help with maintaining your bone density.

Another difficulty for many entering middle age is type 2 diabetes. This occurs when your body reduces its ability to utilize insulin, causing high blood sugar levels. Type 2 diabetes is often preceded by a condition known as insulin resistance. The number of people with type 2 diabetes is on the rise in this country as more and more people become overweight. One of the best ways to keep your blood sugar levels down and help avoid type 2 diabetes is to exercise. When you exercise, your body uses the fuel, the sugar, in your blood to power your activity. In addition, the guidelines on your meal-tracking worksheet make sure that you eat plenty of whole grains, vegetables, and fruits, and minimize the refined sugars and processed foods that contribute to the development of type 2 diabetes. If it hasn't become clear to you yet, using your meal-tracking worksheet and adhering to its guidelines are helping you maximize your health. Think of it as your dietary accountability sheet, helping to keep you lean and active! (Where is yours? Are you using it every day?)

Missing the love boat

Because of the shifting hormones, aging produces a shift in libido. For women, the loss of estrogen can mean vaginal dryness. For men, there can be erection issues. Sexual intimacy is God's gift to us as husbands and wives. The march of time may produce a diminished frequency, but it doesn't have to mean a loss of intensity. If your sexual relationship with your spouse is suffering because of the effects of aging, I encourage you to do a couple of things. First, cut yourself some slack. Just because your desire isn't as all-consuming as when you were newly married, you're not dead sexually. Make adjustments. Give yourself more time. Secondly, talk with each other about what's happening. Sexual subjects, even between sexual partners, can be difficult to express. Work around those barriers, and be open and honest about what you need. Be willing to hear what your partner needs also.

If you're confronted with a persistent physical issue, see your doctor. Your ability to perform sexually is tied to your general health. Hopefully, one of the benefits of a healthier lifestyle will be a more satisfying sexual relationship with your spouse. Be realistic, but don't let your sexuality capitulate to age. It's a lie of society that the only good sex is young sex. God designed our bodies to be sexually active well into our later years.

Counting sheep

One of the casualties of menopause certainly is sleep. Women report difficulty falling asleep and, once asleep, being awakened by hot flashes and night sweats. Women also take longer to fall asleep and can sometimes have trouble turning off a restless mind. All of this bodes ill for the kind of deep, restorative sleep needed to feel rested, alert, and ready to face the day in the morning.

When you were younger, you could count on falling asleep in a minute, scrunched up on a sofa or the floor. It's not that way anymore. Sleep needs to be prepared for; this is true all the time but more so as you age.

- Your bedroom should be for rest. No televisions or computers or desks or workstations! This is your bedroom, not an auxiliary office.
- Keep the lights and the noise levels low as you prepare for sleep. It is difficult for an overstimulated mind to fall asleep. Transition your physical surroundings to support a more relaxed, calming atmosphere.
- Ramp down your activity level in anticipation of sleep. If you're frantically staying up until midnight to finish a work project, don't expect to just drop off the minute the last page is placed in the presentation notebook.
- Turn off the television a half hour before bed, and read or listen to soft music.
- Watch your intake of fluids after about six o'clock at night, and avoid caffeine.
- As Scripture says in Ephesians 4:26, "do not let the sun go down on your anger" (NASU). If you have a problem that's really bothering you and you can do something about it, take the time to address it to gain some measure of resolution before you go to bed. If it's a problem that simply must wait until morning, give it over to God to guard for you during the night. Then, detach yourself from the issue and rest in Him. Go to sleep with prayer.

- Engage in regular exercise, though not right before you need to go to bed. Give your body a chance to recover and relax. Take a nice, hot shower, and go through your normal sleep preparation.
- Wear comfortable clothing to bed. If you're a women undergoing menopause, wear something that is loose and light and preferably cotton, which as a natural fiber will absorb moisture from hot flashes or night sweats.
- Save sleep for the end of the day. Avoid taking naps during the day as a regular practice. These can disturb the natural wake-sleep cycle and confuse your system as to when it's time to go to bed.

The Age God Designed

Reading over Scripture, I am constantly delighted to see how God uses people of all ages—a seven-year-old Joash, an eighty-year-old Moses, and a ninety-year-old Sarah—to accomplish His will. I personally know many people considered "older" by society who live vital lives for God. Their main concern in life is to be active and engaged with the Lord's work. Rich with a life full of experiences and wisdom gained, they are tremendous spiritual resources. In order to be ready for service, they choose to make healthy choices in their lives about what they do and eat and how they treat their bodies. They want to be ready and able when God calls. Though retired from the nine-to-five scene, they are astonishingly busy doing the Lord's work. They see their age as a culmination and fulfillment of a promise, not as a detriment. To them, gray hair is a crown of splendor, and they wear that crown gracefully and gratefully.

Granted, aging does bring about physical and emotional changes that cannot be completely mitigated or reversed. Yet there is a value to aging, and our verse for this chapter alludes to it. Our culture doesn't acknowledge or promote it, but God Himself does. Those who have a relationship with and a calling from God find a purpose for their lives no matter what their age. I love these words from the Book of Joshua: "So here I am today, eighty-five years old! I am still as strong today as the day Moses sent me out; I'm just as vigorous to go out to battle now as I was then. Now give me this hill country that the LORD promised me that day" (Joshua 14:10–12). Caleb didn't bemoan his age. Rather, his focus was on God's promises for his life going forward.

God likewise has promises for your life, promises He is able to fulfill in His time regardless of your age. Does aging bring changes? Yes, but those are changes God knows about and has designed into the body He has given you. Trust Him to be able to help you navigate the changes.

> *Lord, I give this day to You. I give my age to You. I thank You for the blessing of my age. Help me to listen to Your voice and not the culture when it comes to value, worth, and age. My desire, Lord, is not for vain beauty or pride. Rather, my desire is to live this life You've given me in a healthy body, ready and able to respond as Your hands and feet and heart in this world. Allow me to see how my age brings me wisdom and brings me closer to You. When I see my gray head in the mirror, let me see the crown of splendor You have placed there through Your Word! Amen.*

Chapter 11

Wearing Your Swimsuit Down the Runway

Charm is deceitful and beauty is vain, but a woman who fears the Lord, she shall be praised. Give her the product of her hands, and let her works praise her in the gates.

—Proverbs 31:30–31, NASU

There aren't too many people who haven't seen a beauty pageant and watched the slender contestants strut down a runway in full view of a crowd of enthralled, envious watchers. This is truly the world's definition of physical beauty and charm. (It's not all about the swimsuit competition; there's also the question-and-answer part at the end.) We'll gladly watch other people engage in this ritual but would never consider doing such a thing ourselves. Man or woman, the thought of "strutting your stuff," exposed in front of so many people, is nauseatingly scary for most of us. Simply put, we would never expose ourselves to such physical scrutiny. Why? Because we know we're not that good looking, and we'd be humiliated by the reactions and comments. Our physical bodies just couldn't stand up to that kind of exposure.

If we're that fearful of exposing our physical attributes, how do we feel about exposing our spiritual attributes? How would we look in a spiritual swimsuit?

Our True Shape in God: Godliness

Up to this point, I've been talking about the body God designed, and it's been about your physical body. Yes, I've highlighted the fact that your physical body houses an amazing spiritual treasure, but you've really been focusing in on your flesh-and-blood body—what you eat, what you drink, what you do. After all, that's where you're living right now, and that's what you have to contend with. Achieving the body God designed for you is a major step in discovering your true shape in God, but there's more to it than just your physicality.

The best part of this adventure is the true destination of all of this work and sacrifice and learning and understanding. The whole reason to achieve the body God designed is so that you can declare victory over your preoccupation with the physical and really rev your spiritual engine. Listen to Paul's reminder in 1 Timothy 4:8: "For physical training is of some value, but godliness has value for all things, holding promise for both the present life and the life to come."

Do you realize that all this time you've been engaged in training for your physical body you've been learning about godliness, too? You've been multitasking in the best sense of the word. Let's take a quick look back and review what you've learned.

God's intimacy

In reading this book, you were reminded that God made you individually as a one-of-a-kind creation. Through this, you learned the *intimacy* of God's relationship with you. God didn't just create "people," the vast billions and billions who have ever lived; He created you individually. Through His will, He designed a body just for you and nobody else. God knows you intimately, in ways you don't even know yourself. Because of this intimacy, you are learning to trust Him with your struggles about weight and health, as well as about the other challenges you have in life.

God's acceptance

Our journey has reminded you that God is a God of diversity and expansive creativity through all of the different shapes and sizes and styles of bodies He created. Through this, you learned the *acceptance* of God for who you are right now. God is not some captain of a divine softball team, choosing which "players" He wants and doesn't want from a global lineup. God doesn't play favorites. He doesn't choose only the "attractive" people to use in His kingdom. If you doubt that's true (especially after watching some of the well-coiffed, practically-perfect-in-every-way televangelists), consider the description of Jesus written down by the Old Testament prophet Isaiah: "He had no beauty or majesty to attract us to him, nothing in his appearance that we should desire him" (Isaiah 53:2). By worldly standards, Jesus would have been chosen last. But as God often does, He throws our expectations a curveball and makes Jesus first.

God throws us a curveball so we'll understand the world's ways are not His ways. The world may not accept who you are (*you* may not accept who you are), but God does. He's not interested in your six-pack abs or your firm behind unless your preoccupation with them compromises your spiritual growth. His acceptance of you is about who you ultimately are on the *inside*. And as your inside becomes transformed slowly by godliness, your outside will reflect that change.

God's provision

I explained that God designed your body so that it would respond to the physical world in which it has been placed. Through this, you learned about the *provision* of God. You are a spiritual being, yes, but you exist for a time here on this earth in your physical body. Just as Colossians 2:17 describes the law as being a shadow of things to come, your life on Earth here and now is a shadow of what God has in store for you in the future. But His provision and care for you is not relegated to "the sweet by-and-by" alone; God placed you in a physical body in a physical world, and He has designed your body to operate within the world He created. He has made provision for you in this life today.

Sovereignty

I've discussed the fact that God has set up natural consequences for your behavior while you are in your body. Through this, you learned the *sovereignty* of God. You've seen how society has twisted and altered what God intended for your body, especially through the foods you are tempted to eat and the lifestyles you are told to adopt. Your choices have consequences. Positive choices, decisions that take into account the body God designed for you, will produce positive consequences, while negative choices that have more to do with what you want than what you need will have negative consequences. It's your body, but it's God's rules.

There isn't any part of your life that God is not concerned about. When your choices compromise His creation, it becomes His business. When your rebellion over physical things indicates a spiritual rebellion, that's His business, too. You need to learn to trust and obey His rules and submit to His sovereignty in your life. One way you can learn this lesson is through your food and fitness choices.

God's wisdom

I also covered the fact that people tend toward extremes in their desire to attain self-righteousness and perfection. Through this, you learned the *wisdom* of God and of doing things God's way. As an added bonus, you've seen how the thoughts of mankind are foolishness when stacked up to God's wisdom. Our foolishness contributes to our physical conditions, and then we compound that foolishness by trying to "fix" ourselves through extremes.

God instead wants you to be transformed through a process of obedience. Slow and steady wins this race as you consistently turn over to God your challenges and struggles with your weight and body.

God's majesty

Throughout this book, you discovered how intricately and beautifully God has designed your body. Through this you learned the *majesty* of God. Living in the Pacific Northwest, I'm daily reminded of the many beautiful sights in this world, from the waters of Puget Sound to the regal Mount Rainier. They can blind me to the amazing wonders God has designed in something much nearer—my own body.

It's important to see yourself and your body as a creation of God with the same majestic attributes as the mightiest mountain or stunning vista. You reflect God's majesty; wear it proudly.

God's freedom

You read about how easy it is to take a gift of God and use it for selfish gratification. Through this you learned the facets of God's *freedom*. He gave you the freedom to choose to enjoy what He's created within His parameters or choose to hijack those pleasures for selfish gratification. You were not created as a dietary robot who will automatically turn aside from doughnuts and choose broccoli. Instead, you must make choices about what you eat, how much you eat, and why you eat. God desires for you to say yes to Him through your choices, but He gives you the freedom to say no as well.

The question then becomes, what is your response to this freedom? If you can eat doughnuts for breakfast, lunch, and dinner, should you?

I think Paul's response from Romans 6:15 should be your response: "By no means!" The New American Standard Version Updated translates it, "May it never be." Your freedom should not lead you to indulge in poor choices but to acknowledge and follow God all the more willingly and with an obedient heart.

God's comfort

You now know how easy it is for food to be used as a companion, friend, lover, and substitute for God in your life. Through this you've learned the depth of God's *comfort*. Food is a quick fix in the comfort department. It's a microcosm of your life. Comfort from food is like a mist that appears for a little while and then vanishes. (See James 4:14.) The comfort of food doesn't last because it's not built upon anything lasting. When you're lonely, angry, frustrated, hurt, bored, frightened, or anxious, God wants you to turn to Him for comfort, not to food. This is true, lasting, life-changing comfort of the soul, not cheap, quick, instant comfort of the stomach.

God's jealousy

I've shown you how food can become an idol in your life. Through this you learned God's *jealousy*. He will not allow any idols to interfere in your relationship with Him.

Idolatry is a love relationship. It's not such a stretch for you to understand how money can be an idol in your life (2 Timothy 3:2), and you know that the love of money is the root of all kinds of evil (1 Timothy 6:10). But it's harder to accept that about, say, pizza. But just as you can be a lover of money, you can be a lover of food. Either one can become an idol, and neither one is an acceptable substitute for God.

God is jealous to have a love relationship with you, and He does not want to share you with anyone—or anything—else. "For I, the LORD your God, am a jealous God" (Exodus 20:5). Jesus says it this way in Matthew 6:24, which I want you to read in context to your relationship with food: "No one can serve two masters. Either he will hate the one and love the other, or he will be devoted to the one and despise the other."

Whom are you devoted to? Are you serving two masters?

God's peace

I discussed how this fast-paced, hectic world can leave you frazzled, frustrated, and fat. Through this you learned the value of God's *peace*. If you use food as a way to drown out the chaos of your life, try turning down the noise and listening to God so that you can experience His peace instead. His peace eliminates your need for food as stress reliever. As a result, you lose excess weight. Less excess weight means even more peace.

God's plan

In the last chapter, you began to accept that there is a natural process to aging. Through this you learned of God's *plan* for your life. This plan includes the fact that you will continue to age as long as you are alive. Accepting the fact of aging means accepting God's will for your body and for your life.

Now, there's nothing wrong with an attitude like Caleb's. In fact, I hope that when I'm eighty-five years old, I will be as vital and as focused on God's promises as he was! But I want you to accept yourself as you age. Accepting your age is different from fighting against it. God has a plan for you as you age, and it doesn't include trying to look twenty years younger than you are. That's retro thinking, and it binds you to your past and blinds you to the future God holds for you.

Swimsuits Down the Runway

The goal in attaining the body God designed for you is not to wear a slinky swimsuit down a beauty pageant runway. But in the course of my work, I've seen something similar happen. I've seen people who have lost weight successfully. For a few of them, an odd thing happens when they lose the weight. For a time, they revert back to the age they were when they started gaining the weight in the first place. I've seen men in their forties and fifties go out and join much younger local sports teams or start to look around for younger wives. I've seen women in their thirties, forties, and fifties begin to dress like teenagers all of a sudden. It's as if they're going back and reliving something they weren't able to do at the time because of their weight.

A little of this behavior is understandable, but it concerns me when it continues. I'm concerned they'll spend so much time trying to recapture the past that they'll miss out on the present. The body God designed for you is a gift of God meant for today. It's not meant as a way to make up for the past. The past is gone. All you've really been promised is today.

No, the body God designed for you is not meant for a *physical* runway; it is meant for a *spiritual* one. Remember 1 Timothy 4:8, which says, "For physical training is of some value, but godliness has value for all things, holding promise for both the present life and the life to come." You've been in training throughout this book, and it's training that will continue as you solidify into practice the lessons you've learned. It's physical training, but it helps teach you spiritual lessons.

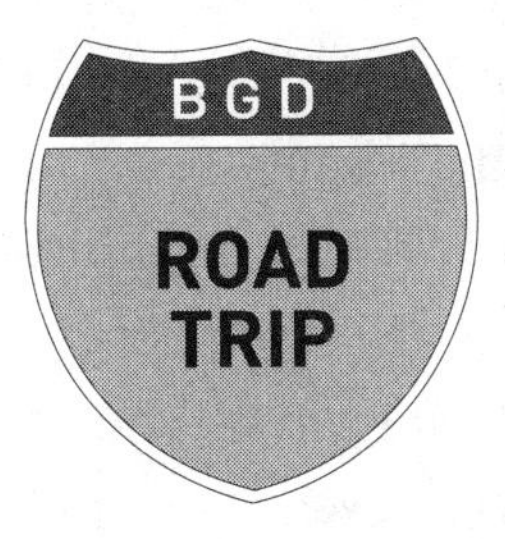

I'd like you to meditate on the 1 Timothy passage that I just quoted. Write down all the ways that physical training has value. Your list could include qualities such as goal setting, perseverance, discipline, self-control, and consistency. Your commitment to regain and maintain the body God designed for you will involve the same traits. Adopting a healthier lifestyle is a kind of physical training. An athlete's training is valuable for a physical event. Your training, however, is for life. It is valuable both here and now and in the hereafter.

Take a moment and write down what you've learned and are learning about your body, yourself, and God through this process. When you need the courage and motivation to continue your commitment, remember these things. When you're starting to beat yourself up because of how far you still have to go, look back and appreciate how far you've come.

You Look Marvelous!

As good as you're looking physically, you're looking even more *fabulous* spiritually! Why? Because all of these lessons you're learning physically have a spiritual application! You are a whole person—emotional, relational, physical, and spiritual. Improvements in one realm strengthen all the others. You may not ever walk down a physical runway, but the lessons you learn from *The Body God Designed* will get you in shape for the spiritual runway. Ultimately, that's the only runway that counts.

We've talked about baby steps on this road to health. A time will come when these habits and choices will no longer be baby steps; they'll become a part of who you are and how you approach food and fitness. After all, we were never meant to be babies forever (as Paul reminds us in 1 Corinthians 3). So, keep taking those baby steps, and become stronger every day. You're coming into your spiritual stride!

Life Is More Than Food

Remember the words of Jesus in Matthew 6:25: "Is not life more important than food?" That's the verse I'd like to leave you with. Because you've taken the time to work through this book, I would venture to guess that your life *has* been all about food. And recently, it's been about changing habits and making choices and cleaning out cupboards and writing down what you eat. It's been about confessing your relationship with food to God and giving it over to Him. It's been about looking at yourself in the mirror and seeing who you really are, not just how you really look.

I applaud your courage. I cannot tell you the number of people I see every day who are trapped in their enmeshment with food and their bodies. I feel their despair. But I also know the freedom that can come through surrendering their lives—including their food—to God.

It is my fervent hope that you've tasted some of God's freedom through this book and you're beginning to recognize and build upon the victories God has given you as you've submitted your eating habits to Him. I understand you may not have "arrived." But I want you to recognize the victories you've had along the way. Now build on those victories. The more entrenched these issues are for you, the more baby steps you'll need to practice until you can walk strong.

Above all, please recognize that God loves you. And if He can love you, you can love yourself. Loving God and being loved by God is more important than food. So, don't try to shortchange or shortcut this training you're in. The work you're doing here is going to reap tremendous spiritual rewards beyond the physical value it has for you. So don't give up!

Don't be disappointed if you haven't gotten as far or gone as fast as you may have wanted. Keep going; have faith!

Don't spend your energy coming up with excuses for why this won't work. Keep going; have faith!

Don't dwell on your failure. Instead, thank God for your victories. Keep going; have faith!

Don't listen to the voices that tell you all this doesn't really matter. It does. Keep going; have faith!

Don't beat yourself up over the past, but recommit yourself to today. Keep going; have faith!

Father God, I'm amazed at what You've done for me so far on this journey to health. Today, I recommit myself to Your wisdom revealed to me along our way together. I acknowledge I need You beside me every baby step of the way. I trust You to allow me to progress down this runway of life, becoming stronger in my walk with You. Thank You for knowing I would need physical help to understand Your spiritual lessons. Thank You that I am learning and using both. I want my body to be the body You created for me. Use it, Lord, for Your glory! Amen.

NOTES

Chapter 2
Hint: The Garden Was Outdoors

1. Gerald F. Fletcher et al., "Statement on Exercise: Benefits and Recommendations for Physical Activity Programs for All Americans," *Circulation* 94 (1996), 857–862, http://circ.ahajournals.org/cgi/content/full/94/4/857 (accessed July 12, 2007).

2. Petra H. Lahman et al., "Physical Activity and Breast Cancer Risk: The European Prospective Investigation into Cancer and Nutrition," *Cancer Epidemiology, Biomarkers & Prevention* (December 2006), 10.1158/1055–9965.EPI-06-0582, http://cebp.aacrjournals.org/cgi/content/abstract/1055-9965.EPI-06-0582v1 (accessed July 12, 2007).

3. American Heart Association, "Physical Activity: AHA Scientific Position," http://www.americanheart.org/presenter.jhtml?identifier=4563 (accessed July 13, 2007).

4. BUPA Health Information Team, "Physical Activity," August 2007, http://hcd2.bupa.co.uk/fact_sheets/html/exercise.html (accessed July 13, 2007).

Chapter 3
Doughnuts: The New Forbidden Fruit

1. Crisco.com, "History and Timeline," http://www.Crisco.com/about/history/index.asp (accessed October 1, 2007).

2. W. C. Willett et al., "Intake of Trans Fatty Acids and Risk of Coronary Heart Disease Among Women," *Lancet* 341 (1993): 581–585, referenced in Harvard School of Public Health, "Fats and Cholesterol: The Good, the Bad, and the Healthy Diet" http://www.hsph.harvard.edu/nutritionsource/fats.html (accessed October 4, 2007).

3. University of Sydney, "About Glycemic Index," http://www.glycemicindex.com (accessed October 1, 2007).

Chapter 4
My Kingdom for Some Chromium

1. Ronald Kotulak, "Vitamin a Day Just What Doctor Ordered," *Chicago Tribune*, June 19, 2002.

Chapter 5
Fear-o-fat-o-phobia

1. Daniel Woolls, "Models Flunk BMI, Get Spain Fashion Boot," Boston.com, September 8, 2006, http://www.boston.com/news/world/Europe/articles/2006/09/08/models_flunk_BMI_get_spain_fashion_boot/ (accessed October 1, 2007).

2. University of Maryland Center for Integrative Medicine, "Omega-3 Fatty Acids," http://www.umm.edu/altmed/articles/omega-3-000316.htm (accessed July 16, 2007).

3. This information on omega-6s is also from the University of Maryland Medical Center for Integrative Medicine. It is found in an article called, "Omega-6 Fatty Acids," http://www.umm.edu/altmed/articles/omega-6-000317.htm (accessed July 16, 2007).

Chapter 7
The Proper Use of the Knife

1. PBS.org, "Bariatric Surgery: Quick Facts," http://www.pbs.org/secondopinion/episodes/bariatricsurgery/quickfacts/index.htm (accessed October 1, 2007).

2. CNN.com, "Poll: Most Americans Older Than 25 Are Overweight," March 5, 2002, http://www.pbs.org/secondopinion/episodesbariatricsurgery/quickfacts/index.html (accessed October 1, 2007).

3. Grete Waitz, "Exercise Is Life," JP Morgan Chase Corporate Challenge, http://www.jpmorganchasecc.com/07grete/gtfitlife.htm (accessed October 1, 2007).

4. Ibid.

5. Denise Grady, "Diabetes Rises; Doctors Foresee a Harsh Impact," *New York Times*, August 24, 2000, http://query.nytimes.com/gst/fullpage.html?res=9F04E5DD1431F937A1575BC0A9669C8B63 (accessed October 1, 2007).

6. McDonalds.com, "McDonald's USA Nutrition Facts for Popular Menu Items," http://www.mcdonalds.com/app_controller.nutrition.index1.html (accessed April 1, 2007).

7. For example, Calorie Count from About.com Health: http://www.calorie-count.com/calories/browse/1900.html..

Chapter 9
Be Still and Know that I Am Chocolate

1. There is a great deal of useful, general information on stress to be found online at www.webmd.com. While not particularly comprehensive, it's a good overview and is worth looking over.

2. WebMD.com, "Effects of Stress," Stress Management Health Center, http://www.webmd.com/balance/tc/Stress-Management-Effects-of-Stress (accessed July 19, 2007).

Chapter 10
I'll Take the Crown but Not the Gray

1. WebMd.com, "Menopause Not Just for Women," October 24, 2001, http://men.webmd.com/features/menopause-not-just-for-women (accessed July 19, 2007)

Index

A

B

C

D

E

R

S

T

U